CHRONIC PAIN AND ME

RICHARD N SCOTT

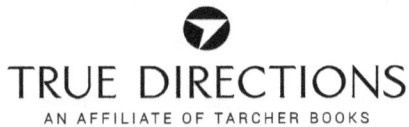

TRUE DIRECTIONS
AN AFFILIATE OF TARCHER BOOKS

CHRONIC PAIN AND ME

iUniverse books may be ordered through booksellers or by contacting:

iUniverse
1663 Liberty Drive
Bloomington, IN 47403
www.iuniverse.com
1-800-Authors (1-800-288-4677)

ISBN: 978-1-4917-3305-9 (sc)
ISBN: 978-1-4917-3306-6 (hc)
ISBN: 978-1-4917-3307-3 (e)

Library of Congress Control Number: 2014907552

Printed in the United States of America.

iUniverse rev. date: 08/01/2014

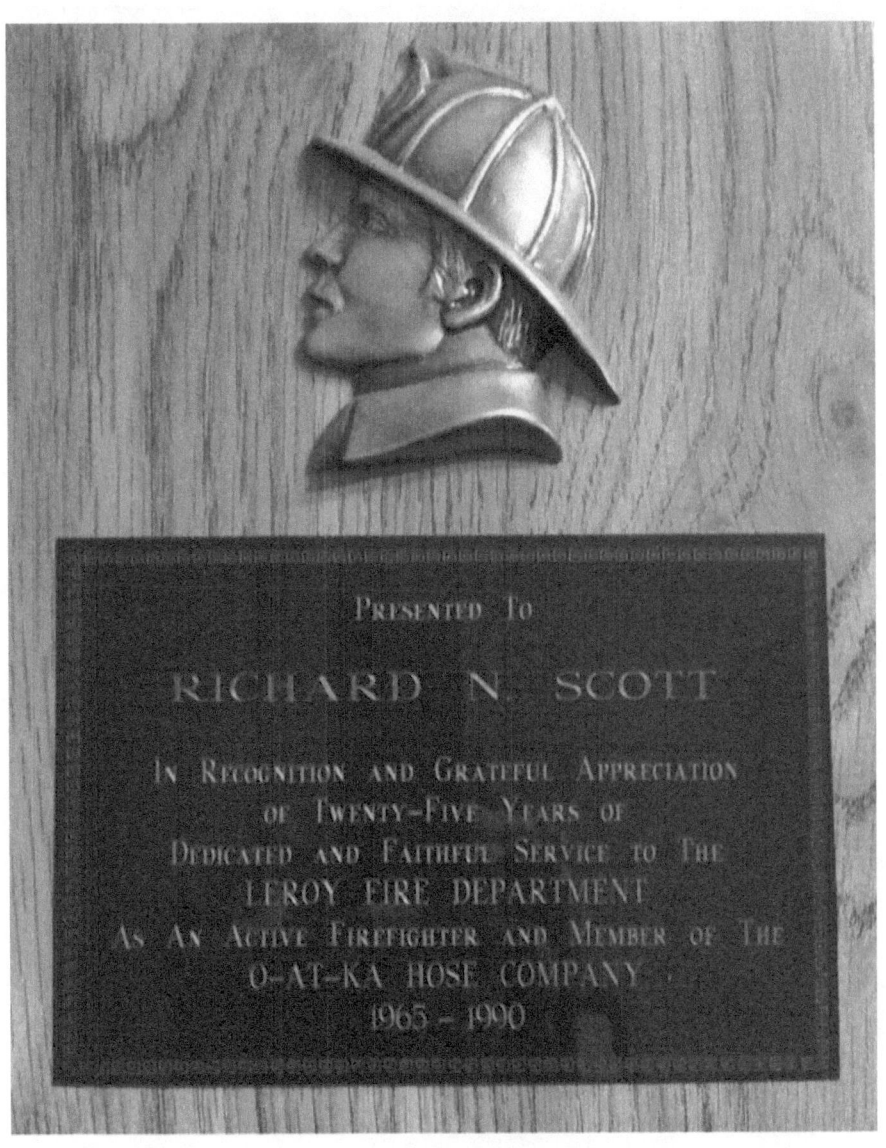

This award was for over twenty years of service as a volunteer firefighter.

I wanted to give back to my community ==

To Connie Chiler Scott

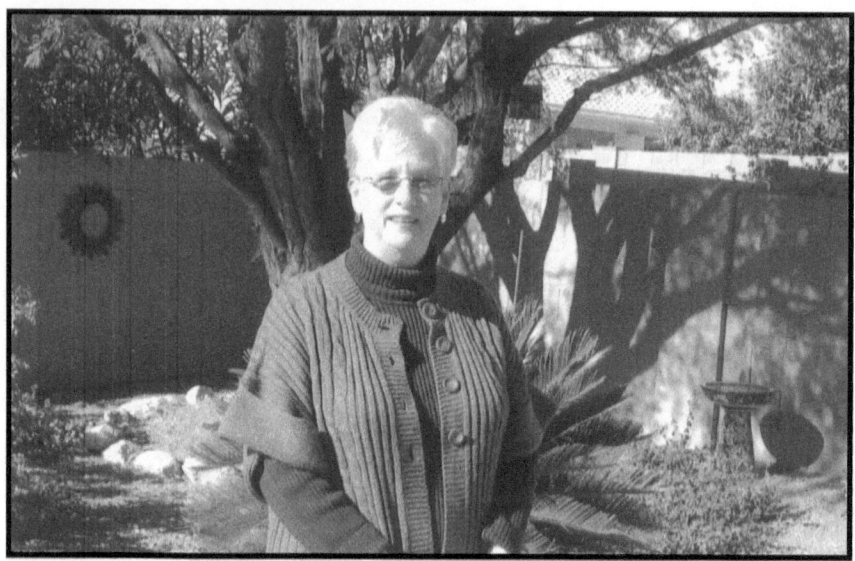

My loving wife of more than forty-five years took care of me for more than eleven years, giving me constant care. She dedicated her life to me and the injuries that I sustained from a terrible fall in October 2000. Connie gave me the inspiration, courage, and fortitude to write this autobiography of my life since I was hurt. This book took me almost four years to complete, and unfortunately, I lost this love of my life on February 25, 2012. She was loved by many people and held the position of a registered nurse, which she dedicated her life to.

Connie was the daughter of Corrin and Helen graham Chiler. She was also the daughter-in-law to Willis and Rose Bean Scott

To our special daughter, Jennifer Lynne Scott

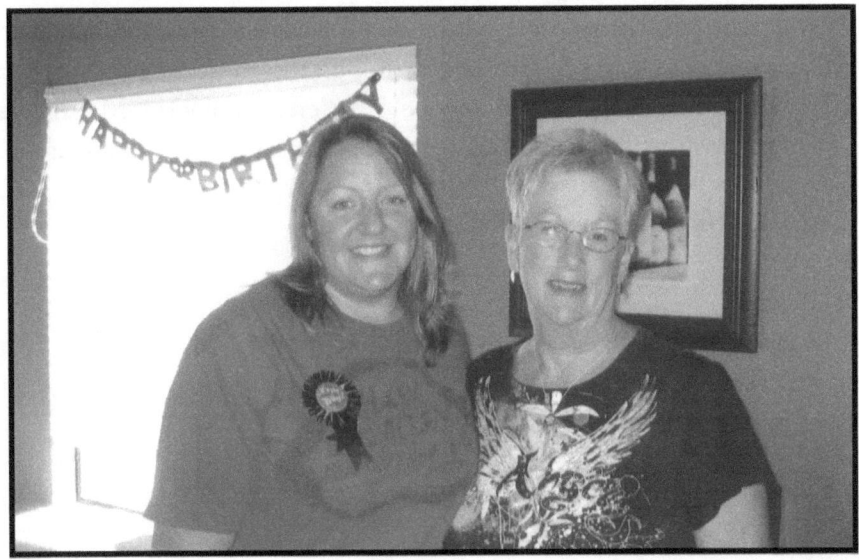

On February 19, 1971, Connie and I were blessed with the most beautiful child God could have ever sent to us. This baby was the answer to our dreams, and we finally had a family, which we had tried so long for.

Jennifer was by far the best thing that ever happened to us, and we made sure that this wonderful daughter would never be short on love. Our families embraced this bundle of joy, and they knew that our family was now complete with the addition of Jenny.

As time went on, Jenny surprised us all by deciding to become a registered nurse just like her mother. She wore her shoes well and has become an outstanding nurse in her field. Jenny and Connie were very close, and their bond was as strong at the end as it was when it was created.

Jenny, you are the best of the best, and we love you so.

Additional Special Recognition

During these past thirteen-plus years, I have dealt with many people who have given me the help I needed to get through this most devastating time in my life. If I have overlooked anyone, I sincerely apologize. My sincere thanks and love go out to all of these people who cared so much about me.

In Batavia, New York, and Buffalo, New York:
Dr. Mir
Dr. Bagnall
In Le Roy , New York, at Le Roy Physical Therapy:
Pat Privitera and staff
All of my close friends to numerous to mention

In Rochester, New York:
Dr. Zeidman
Dr. Nemani

In Arizona:
Dr. Martin E. Weinand the doctor that changed my life
Dr. Carolyn
Dr. Katz
Dr. Hasler
Dr. Tsau
Dr. Goldsmith
Dr. Greenberg
Dr. Mark A Strumpf & Arlene Bahr
Josh Reddoch and Riley Post (whom I will never forget)
Win Tandy--He has the knowledge of the computer
All of my close friends to numerous to mention

At St. Jude Medical:
Travis Heckler
Denise Landry

I would not have survived without my daughter, Jennifer Lynne Scott; my sisters, Elaine Scott Pike and Sharon Scott Collins; and all of my nieces and nephews. In many ways, they dedicated themselves to me at times to keep me from deep depression and anxiety so I could keep forging ahead. My family is everything to me and always will be.

My God above has helped me to handle the problems, of which, I thoughtwere ever possible. I have dedicated my life to my God and my very loving family all over the United States.

PREFACE

My life with intense chronic pain for several years had motivated me to write a book detailing everything I faced during my thirteen years of hell and frustration. I have great hope that anyone reading this book who also deals with chronic pain will find alternatives to the very painful life they are living with today.

CHAPTER 1

I was born in September 1945 to Willis and Rose Scott. I was about to begin a life that I never would have expected—a life of pain, which would start when I was five years old. The different things that happened to me over the years would never be put into a book until I was fifty-five years old and had faced the hardest and most destructive pain I would ever face in my life. It is chronic pain that never stops, and you live or die with it.

Early in my life, when I was about five years old, I was riding my tricycle when I fell over on my handlebar. The handlebar had no handgrip on it and pushed very hard into my stomach cavity. What first was very painful quickly subsided to where the pain had gone away completely. I told no one of my fall, as I didn't want my mom to get mad.

A few days later my father and brother-in-law were playing with me in the front yard and began throwing me back and forth when I let out a very painful scream. My dad immediately laid me on the ground and hollered for my mother, who came running out of the door. I was lying on the ground crying uncontrollable, and my dad told my mother what had happened. She immediately picked me up carefully, took me to the backseat of the car, and gently laid me down. My sister had come out of the house with a pillow and a blanket, and before I knew it, we were on the way to the hospital twenty minutes away.

Pulling into the parking lot near the emergency room, my dad hurriedly got out of the car and went to the backseat. He cradled me in his arms and carried me into the hospital entrance. When we got inside, my mother explained what had happened earlier in the day, and a doctor soon showed up and began to check me over. He had felt my stomach area, and I hollered out in intense pain. He made the decision to have an x-ray taken right away. After seeing the results, they prepared me for immediate surgery, as they had seen a problem that had to be corrected.

In about an hour, I was under the knife, and they immediately discovered that I had a cyst on my pancreas. I was operated on and back in the recovery room inside of four hours. The doctor told my mother that I had gone through a very serious surgery, and the outcome should be known in the next few hours. I was taken first to recovery for a period of time. When I was back in my room, I was still groggy. When I was able to communicate, my mom began asking me questions, because she had no idea how this problem had originated. I told her that I had fallen on my bike the day before and explained how at first it hurt quite a bit but soon after my fall the pain went away and I started playing again. So this is how all of a sudden I became so sick. My mom told me to always tell her if I ever got hurt so she would know, and I told her I would.

I was able to return home in about a week with strict orders to rest—no rough stuff. I was lying on the couch the second day home and just relaxing when an awful pain came from my stomach area again, and I began screaming. I was immediately put into the car and rushed to the hospital. This time, a call was made to advise the hospital that I was on the way. When we arrived, people were waiting for me at the emergency room door. I was rushed right to surgery.

My doctor happened to be in the hospital at the time and had me immediately prepared for surgery. After the surgery, which took about another three to four hours, I was sent to the recovery room until I felt well enough to go back to my room. When I was taken back to my room, my mom was there with tears streaming from her eyes and very upset. My doctor soon walked in, and they both went into the hall. He told my mom that I had a bowel obstruction and was very fortunate to have gotten to the hospital as quickly as I did. He mentioned that I was given a brand-new drug called penicillin, and I was the first one in the area to use it. My name was eventually placed in a medical journal for being the youngest patient with this type of problem to have been treated with penicillin.

With the two surgeries came many steel staples to stitch up the openings in my stomach. When I was finally released to go home, I had very strict orders on what I could and could not do. It would take many weeks for my scars to heal, and I had to be very quiet. I had to return to the hospital in a couple of weeks to have the staples removed. For the balance of the summer, there was no more rough stuff outside.

I was able to sleep on a couch downstairs and would not be able to go out to play for a long time. I had visitors who came to see me on a regular basis. These operations prevented me from playing football or any other rough activities in the future

As time went on, I was to face a new pain that resulted from the surgeries I had at only five years old. I began having adhesions when I was ten years old which were gas pockets that formed around the scar tissue from my surgeries. At times, I would be rushed to the hospital with intense pain due to my stomach bloating up with gas. In the hospital, I would have to have a tube put down my nose and into my stomach to suck out anything in my stomach and release the gas pockets. I continued having these gas pockets until I was about sixteen years old. Along with the gas pockets, I had a very bad problem trying to go to the bathroom. My problem was constipation, and the only way the problem would be eliminated was by taking mineral oil every other day so I could go to the bathroom. This continued for many years until I was twenty years old, when I was able to stop taking the "motor oil."

After those two operations, I ended up at home for a couple of months before I could go back to first grade. This resulted in me being held back one year. I had to learn how to walk again, as well as other things due to me having to rest and not do anything that could create a problem as a result of my surgeries. Due to these major surgeries, the scars on my stomach were very large, completely encompassing my whole stomach. I became very self-conscious of my appearance when I would go swimming, as everyone would continually stare at my stomach. This affected me mentally. It bothered me so much that I would not go swimming unless I went with my parents or sisters, and they helped me get through this very tough problem. This went on for many years until I finally just let it slide. It actually looked like I had three belly buttons, and in fact, this is what friends would say to me.

As I kept growing and made my way through life, I would have my scrapes and falls but nothing ever big enough to land me back into the hospital. One of the very hard things for me to handle was that I was unable to play football. The doctors' reasoning was that any hard blows to my stomach may kill me. All of my close friends were playing, and I was on the sidelines. So I began playing basketball to get my mind off of this very hard thing for me. I practiced all of the time. Regardless of the weather, I played all of the time.

When basketball season came around, I tried out for the junior varsity team and was very happy to be selected to play. I had really worked hard for my first year when I was unable to play football. The harder I worked, the better I got. Unfortunately, I was about five nine, which was pretty short, and I couldn't jump like I really wanted too. Going through my freshman year, I played in almost every game until the end of the season when I was asked to move up to the varsity team. I had gotten to know the varsity coach very well, and one day he asked me to come to his apartment house to move some furniture for him. A friend and I went there and found we had to move a refrigerator up two flights of stairs for him.

The coach had brought in a two-wheel cart, and we began the move. As we were moving the appliance up the stairs, the appliance suddenly shifted. I lunged at it and felt my back snap. The friend who was on top of the appliance asked me if I was okay, and I said yes. We continued on until we finished the job. The coach thanked us, and we left for home. When I got home, I felt a pain in my back that I'd never had before. My dad had a very bad back and some nights I would have to get on the floor with him to rub his back. I hoped that I would not end up like that a few years down the road. Through the night, my back began to hurt a little more.

When I woke up the next morning, the pain was very bad, and I was actually hunched over. I could not straighten up. The harder I tried, the worse it became. I didn't know what to do, because I wasn't sure I could go to school in my condition. I finally decided that I would have to deal with the pain if I wanted to go to school. When I was getting ready, my sister said something to me about my back, but I really didn't hear what she said. I had not told anyone what I had done at the coach's house. I knew that in school I would be kidded, but when I got home that night, there would be fifty questions. I went to school and was really kidded all day long. When I sat down in a hard chair, my back became much worse.

I had been looking at this girl in school for quite some time. I had talked with her many times, but I really was interested. I wondered what she would say when she saw me. I decided that I couldn't worry about that, as my back was really bad and there wasn't anything I could do. I finally made it through the day. When I got home, I was really hunched over, and the fifty questions began. My dad asked me what had happened, and I told him. He had told me so many times to take care of my back. He had hurt his many years earlier and suffered every day with his. He had awful pain. I realized that it looked like I had really screwed up and hurt mine. My dad told me that it would likely get worse unless I took care of it right away. The pain was bad enough that I was still all hunched over. I decided that I would wait and see what happened the next morning. There were no more comments from the family that night, as I am sure my dad told them I already felt bad enough.

I woke up the next morning and really hurt very bad. I knew that I could not make it to school but needed to get to the doctor. I waited for the time they opened, and my mom took me to the doctor. He was a friend and sympathized with me. He gave me a prescription for valium to take when needed. We went and got the prescription filled and went home. I took one and felt much better a few hours later. As the day went on, I kept getting better until I went to bed. When I got up the next day, I felt fine. I really took it easy and put my valium in the kitchen cupboard for a later date. It looked like I could get through this if I really was careful in what I did.

I sure didn't want the pain to get any worse, so I had to be really careful with my back/.

Over the months, I would have problems every once in a while but it looked like I could handle it if I watched what I was doing. When I played basketball, I had some problems a couple of times but was able to get through it. The pills I had would last me a long time if I was careful.

I got through my sophomore year, and my back went out on me twice. I had to use the valium and take it easy, and then it would straighten out again so I would be back to normal. Soon it became evident that each time my back went out the pain became much worse. I began to worry about what was going to happen. I just continued doing everything I liked and was doing fine.

During my junior year, my back seemed to be doing pretty good. I really watched what I did very carefully. I had shop class every day and liked the class and the instructor. One particular day I went to class, and we were working on a project being made from steel. I was working with a milling machine, which cut very small pieces off a larger piece of steel when it passed over it. I had been getting filings off of the piece I was cutting, and they were hitting my arm and burning it. I didn't have a long-sleeved shirt on, so I decided to put on a pair of welder's gloves. This is not recommended when working with this machine, but I felt I would be very careful. While I was working, someone called me from across the room, and I took my eyes off of the machine to look toward the area where the voice came from. At that moment, I felt an awful pain in my hand. I looked down and saw my index finger being pulled through the cutting blades of the machine. I tried to stop the machine, but it finally stopped on its own. Evidently, the belt had slipped, as my finger was too big to pass through. I turned the machine on again and put it into reverse. The glove came out of the machine, and when I pulled my hand out, the top of my index finger fell to the floor. A friend saw what had happened and rushed over to me to put his handkerchief over my hand. The blood was spurting out of the end of my index finger.

My friend screamed to the shop instructor. When he approached the area, he saw my finger on the floor and became very woozy. He picked the finger up, placed it in his hanky, and gave it to my friend who was going to rush me to the hospital. It took us twenty minutes to get there, and there was a surgeon on hand to take care of the reattachment. It took about an hour or so, and I was all stitched up with fifty stitches. He then wrapped my finger and hand, and I was instructed not to use the finger at all.

Friday night came, and I was put into the game before it was over. On Saturday morning, I was back to the hospital to have my finger stitched up again. For the next few days, the pain from my healing finger was very intense. It continually throbbed, and I couldn't sleep or do anything else, including playing basketball. I had to wait three months before I was able to play again. We only had one game left in the season, but that was okay.

The girl that I was sweet on was going to graduate the following year, and I was a year behind her because of my early surgeries in my life. We began seeing each other, and it was very serious. She was going to nursing school, and I was going to be a senior in high school. As time went by, I had to live with my back the way it was, as I was not going to have anyone touch it. My dad had been suffering with his back issues for years, and his life was definitely not very good with all of the pain he had to live with. I would still rub his back on nights when it was really bothering him.

The girl I really liked who's name was Connie Chiler, and she lived in Le Roy. She was a few months older than I was and lived only about ten minutes from our house via car. She decided to go to college in Rochester, New York, at a nursing school. She had wanted to be a nurse for a long time, and I was sure she would be a good one. While she was in her second year of school, we became engaged and planned to get married in August of 1966 Up to that point, I had already faced much pain and many problems with my body. I'd had to spend quite a bit of time in the hospital and was very use to having shots. I had to be tough, and I was. The stomach problem would eventually prevent me from being drafted into the US Armed Forces. My stomach was so tender that any hard blow could kill me, so I had to be really careful the rest of my life with regard to the things I did.

My back had been good and bad through my senior year in high school. I wasn't sure what I was going to do after graduating, but I was almost sure I would not be attending college. I wished I was, but I was very much in love with Connie and wanted to get married.

I graduated from high school in 1964, and Connie graduated from college in 1965. After graduation, I went to work with a company in Batavia, and my back was really bothering me by this point in time. I could not be any easier on my back, but I was really worried what the outcome was going to be.

CHAPTER 2

in 1966, Connie and I were married. Connie went to work at the local hospital, and we lived in an apartment. My back continued to get worse, and then I had another pain that took me over. I found the pain to be kidney stones. I have had so many different types of pain since I was born. Each pain has been different. With all of the pain that I have had to deal through the years, I have learned that all pain is different. It affects you differently. In all of my experiences with pain, I can say that the kidney stones have definitely been the worst pain I have ever experienced. There's no mistake; nothing has been worse. I ended up having kidney stones—and all the pain that goes with them—nine times. I have had much more pain in my nearly seventy years of life than most people will ever have in their lives. I sure hope that I am all done, as I feel that I have had my fair share.

I do not remember how painful my stomach operations were, but my mother told me I cried an awful lot. I do remember the pain from my back when I hurt it. When it was bad, it was pretty intense, and sitting down really hurt me an awful lot. When I cut my finger off, another type of pain was created, which was very bad at times. These injuries really had to make me very tough. The next thing I faced was kidney stones. I couldn't even begin to tell anyone how bad that pain is. You can never find a position that relieves the pain. The pain is always there until the stone is gone. Now, about my back problem. My back is really getting very painful. Living with this in 1978 I don't know how much longer I can hold out .

I am now working for a corrugated box company in 1986. . The pain was really beginning to get very bad and I was glad that I also still had the Valium that the doctor prescribed to me back in 1963, more than twenty years earlier. I drove to work one morning, and my back was really giving me trouble. I made it to about ten o'clock that morning and then had to leave work. When I got home, I ended up calling the ambulance, which took me to the hospital. I was immediately taken to surgery. The surgery was a total success. After it was over, I felt great. I hadn't felt that good in more than twenty years. It was unexplainable how good I felt. I was finally all better and hoped that I wouldn't experience any more pain for the rest of my life—I hoped.

It was as if I had been picked by God to handle the ultimate in pain before I left this earth. Connie and I had been through so much up to that point in time, and in October of 2000, the ultimate of injuries hit me with little knowledge in what I was going to have to face over the next ten-plus years.

The company I worked for was having new carpets installed in the upstairs offices. To get to the offices upstairs, you had to go up a steel and concrete staircase. On this particular morning, I arrived to work at about six thirty and had just come off of vacation. I could always get a lot done with no one in the office with me. Soon, the other employees walked through the doors, and the day began. After working around the installers for about three hours, I decided to go to the cafeteria at about ten thirty to get something to eat. I went through a couple of offices, opened the door to the staircase, and put my foot down only to go airborne down the stairs.

I could not believe what had happened to me. Another injury and more pain—I wondered why God was letting this happen to me. What had I done wrong in order to have all of these problems occur in my life? I thought I had been a good individual and a loving person. But I was having so many problems and being hurt so much. I did not know what was in store for me, but I knew that I would have to handle it. I remember thinking to myself: *What will the outcome be this time God? Am I going to be able to handle it? How much pain am I going to have? Will I be able to continue work?* I had thought of all of these questions and was very worried about what would happen to me and my wife. However, I realized that we wouldn't know until a little later in life.

I had to lie on the stairs with someone holding my legs so I wouldn't slide farther down the stairs. My back had hurt, and I'd just had it operated on a few years earlier. My neck also hurt and who knows what else. I asked what had happened to me and found out that the stairs were being prepared for the new carpet to be placed. Glue had been applied to the top ten treads, and that's what I stepped on. There were no warning signs anywhere. I had gobs of glue that stuck to all of my clothes and some on my head. After I was placed on the gurney, before I could be removed from it, my clothes had to be cut off.

The ambulance came to our business to pick me up. They put me on a board and also put a neck brace on me. After all of the procedures, they loaded me into the ambulance. I had some pain in my back and neck but not an awful lot at that point. The trip to the hospital took us about twenty minutes. I was unloaded off of the ambulance and wheeled directly into the emergency room. Nurses came into the cubical and began cutting more of my clothes off, which were stuck to the gurney. The ambulance crew helped move me over to the hospital bed and then left.

I felt the pain beginning to increase at that point. My back was what really began to hurt more. All I could think of was the surgery I'd had in 1986. It had turned out great, and I realized I may be facing something worse this time around. At that point, I had asked the nurse for pain medicine, as I was feeling my back much more. One of the nurses brought in a nightgown for me to put on after all of my clothes were taken off. Then a doctor came in and wrote orders for me to have a full line of tests, including x-rays and other tests, to determine what injuries, if any, I had sustained. The nurse mentioned the pain medicine to the doctor, and he directed her to give me a shot of morphine.

About ten minutes later, the x-ray tech came into the cubical and wheeled me to the x-ray department. Because of my previous back surgery, I had problems lying on the hard x-ray tables, and the pain could become very bad. After getting me in position, they began shooting films. About ten minutes later, that portion of the test were done. A short time later, I was to have an MRI and whatever else they wanted me to have. As I was wheeled back into the emergency room, I saw Connie who had just arrived. She bent over and gave me a kiss. There were no questions in the beginning, as she was just concerned about how I was feeling.

Next, I was taken to have an MRI and was gone from my room for about an hour. After all of the very hard tables, my back was hurting an awful lot. I couldn't wait to get back to that bed. Soon, I was wheeled back to my cubical and into the bed. Connie and I were there talking about what happened, and about an hour later, a doctor came in to release me. He mentioned that there was no sign of damage to my neck or back. He suggested that I go home and relax and see my primary care physician the next day. Connie had gone out to get the car to pick me up at the emergency room parking lot, and I signed out and was wheeled to the parking lot area so we could leave. I was helped into the car, and Connie was on the way to our home in Le Roy.

About an hour after leaving the hospital, we pulled into the driveway at our home. The pain began getting worse in my back, but I had no pain medication from the hospital. Fortunately we had pain medication from other back problems I'd had in the past. After getting situated and lying on the couch, Connie called my doctor and made an appointment for me to see him the next day in Batavia. All of the beds in our home were water beds. I really enjoyed sleeping on this type of bed, but with my neck and back problem, I could not lie on my bed any longer, at least for the time being. Instead, I had to plan on sleeping and resting on the couch in the living room until we figured things out. It became hard for me right away to settle in on the couch, but I knew that it was the only place I could rest and sleep.

The rest of the day was quite slow. My back gradually got worse, but I really didn't have much of a problem with my neck at that time. I tried to watch television, and I would coast off to sleep every once in a while. Finally, I was able to fall asleep for the night, but I had to get up a couple of times during the night to go to the bathroom.

I woke up at about seven o'clock the next morning, and my back hurt quite a bit. My neck had also started hurting a lot. I wondered why I had so much pain in both places despite the fact that they hadn't seen anything in any of the films. I hoped that after seeing my doctor, I would have some idea regarding what route we would take. I was hopeful that I would be able to return to work soon, as we definitely needed the money. I could be off a few weeks to recuperate, but I didn't want to get too far behind. After all, it was my company's problem for having these carpet guys working during business hours. I don't want to say that I knew it was going to happen, but no one was really thinking about what possibly may happen.

The morning went fairly quickly, and we got ready in the afternoon for my doctor's appointment at two thirty. By this time, my neck and back hurt more, and I had hope that I could get some medication to help with the pain. The doctor told me he would give me some pain medication to get through the rough times with my back and neck. He then made out a prescription for us to get filled when we got home. I told him the story of what happened, and he told Connie and me that he was going to refer me to a neurologist. My doctor felt that there wasn't anything he could really do for me and believed I needed to be looked at in much more detail. He gave us the name of another doctor who was also in Batavia. When we got home, we stopped at the pharmacy to get the prescription filled for the pain medication. This would help me much more than what I was already taking. When we got home, Connie called the neurologist's office and made an appointment to see him.

Unfortunately, I started to become somewhat depressed over the whole situation. I couldn't help but wonder what the final outcome of this fall would be. This had happened during a time when I was completely watching what I was doing, but because of some very poor planning on the carpet layers' part, I ended up getting hurt. I didn't even know how bad things were yet, but I knew that I was having pain in my back and fourteen years earlier I'd had a very positive surgery done where everything turned out great. Now I was facing the possibility of having surgery again at some point in time. My neck had not been feeling well either. So many things were going through my mind.

I wondered if I should consider a lawsuit. I didn't know if I should, but I had to make sure to protect myself and Connie should something transpire later on as a result of my fall. I realized I needed to talk to someone about what I should do. I also wondered how long I could be out of work; I knew that I had four weeks of vacation coming up the following year.

I'd been having a slight problem at home sleeping on the couch. After sleeping on the waterbed for so long, it was hard to adjust to such a sudden sleeping arrangement. Connie was very concerned that the waterbed may cause a major problem with my back, and I didn't want to take any chances either. The couch, however, was quite hard for my back as well. My neck was also creating a problem for me, but I knew that there was nothing else to do at that time. I would have to continue to sleep on the couch until other arrangements were made. I had the appointment with the neurologist the following afternoon at three o'clock. I hoped that we would be able to get some answers to everything that was going on.

I woke up at about seven o'clock the next morning and didn't feel too good when I got up. My back hurt, but my neck seemed to be getting worse. Things were really beginning to wear on me, as no one could see anything in any of the films. I was sure the new doctor would want me to have some type of x-rays done or maybe something else. My depression was worse the day of the appointment with the neurologist. Fortunately, I had pills at home that I could take if I got depressed. On that day, I did decide take a Hydrocodone at about noon, as I was really getting uneasy. We would need to leave for the doctor's office at about two thirty, and it would take us about fifteen minutes to get there.

Connie had showered and was getting ready. It was now one o'clock, and it was my turn to take a shower. I got in and showered. My neck continued to hurt, along with my back. I was experiencing a small headache, which I'd never had before the accident. I began to wonder if that was something

I was going to be having a lot more of. With the hard fall I'd had, it was impossible to know. I would just have to wait and see. I got done with the shower and dressed. When I was done, I lay down on the couch and waited for the time to leave.

Connie had finished getting ready and asked if I was ready to go. I told her I had to get my shoes on and go to the bathroom, and then I would be ready. It was kind of chilly out, so I made sure I had my winter coat on. We both got into the car and headed for Batavia for my appointment. It took us about twenty minutes to get to the doctor's office. We pulled into the parking lot and got out of the car. My back was really bothering me, and I had to walk around for about ten minutes to straighten up. Connie had already gone into the office, and I then walked through the door and announced myself.

We took our coats off, and Connie sat in the chair in the waiting room while I stood up and walked around the office. The receptionist then gave me some insurance papers to fill out, which I gave to Connie. She worked on them for a few minutes, and then I signed them and returned them to the girl. I was unable to sit down, as my lower back was very painful. As I paced back and forth, there was another person in the office waiting to see the doctor. Connie whispered to me that I might be annoying the other person with my pacing. I kindly apologized to the lady and told her I was very sorry but I couldn't sit. She told me that I was not bothering her at all and to continue to walk. I know that Connie was very embarrassed about my pacing, but there was nothing I could do, as I could not stand in one spot.

About ten minutes later, we were called into the doctor's office. I introduced Connie and myself to the doctor. He, in turn, introduced himself and then asked what he could do for me. I briefly explained the accident and my meeting with our family doctor. I mentioned that our doctor suggested that I see him about my problems. The doctor examined me and decided that he wanted me to have some x-rays and possibly an MRI at a later date. In the meantime, he wanted me to go to physical therapy twice a week for a few weeks and then return to see him. I agreed to have the x-rays as soon as possible, and then I would start with therapy. He gave me two prescriptions, one for the x-ray and one for the therapy sessions. At that time, I had an idea that I wasn't going to find out what type of problems I had.

My depression was not getting any better, and I didn't know what I was going to do. Connie and I talked about it for a while, and I agreed to see a friend of ours who was a psychologist. When we got home, Connie called our friend Dr. L on the phone to see if he possibly would come to the house to see me. I was not in any shape at that point to go to his office, as I was becoming very discouraged about my internal problems. I really wanted to see him at our home. He agreed to come by and set up a meeting time with Connie. It was going to be a couple of days before I would see Dr. L unless I needed him sooner.

It was at that time that I began to notice another problem I was having. I could not urinate unless I pushed on my stomach for a while. At times, it took me ten minutes to go. Also, trying to have a bowel movement was very odd. When I would get ready to go, I had very little feeling if I was going or not. The way I determined if I had gone was to either get up and look or wait for the relief in my stomach. I realized that I would have to mention these issues to a doctor when I saw one.

I was lying on the couch when Connie got off the phone, and I told her that I would go to the physical therapy office the following day to set up appointments. I really was totally convinced that I should be doing this, but I would try to see what the outcome would be when my therapy was over. Connie also called and set up an appointment for me to go and have x-rays taken of my back and neck.

Lying on the couch, I had the chance to think of many things that were happening to me and Connie. I had forgotten that she would be losing her job with the doctors' office where she worked in February 2001. All the doctors decided to retire or do other things, and Connie would not have a job. This could not have come at a worse time for us. With me out of work and her also out of work, what would we do to pay the bills? I couldn't help but think that something was happening because God was not happy with me for some reason; I just didn't know what it may be. It was at that time when I started to keep a log of my pain and the drugs I was taking. It was a must.

Each time I would think of all of the problems we faced, my depression just became worse. How were we ever going to get through all of this? In any event, we had to. Somehow we would make it through it as we had done in the past.

Just lying there, I fell asleep for about an hour, and then I woke up and had to get ready for dinner. After eating, I decided to lie on the couch, as I didn't feel like doing anything at all. I decided that I would go to sign up at therapy when Connie got up the next morning. I gradually coasted off to sleep and finally woke up at about midnight and had to go to the bathroom. After going to the bathroom, I again fell asleep. Connie was still watching TV.

I woke up at about eight o'clock in the morning, got up, and walked around the house for a few minutes to see how much I hurt. Again, my neck hurt worse than my back. The pain was beginning to be worse, and I knew that I was going to need stronger medication pretty soon. Connie didn't get up until about ten thirty, and by the time she got ready, it was about two thirty. I also got ready, and we drove to the physical therapy office. It was only about ten minutes from our home. We went inside, and I went to sign in. The receptionist had given me a couple of sheets for insurance. Connie took them as usual and filled in all the information. All I did was sign itand continue to walk around.

It was about twenty minutes later when the owner of the facility came over to talk with us for a minute. He explained what he was going to do to hopefully help me out. He basically told us that he would try to help me, but at times, the therapy did not help the person, so other things would have to be tried. I definitely liked this guy as he was very straightforward with us and held nothing back. We had to set up our first appointment to start my therapy. Connie pulled out her appointment book, and a date was set for three days later. My appointments would be twice a week at his building there. We thanked him and left. It was now October 23, 2000, and I was praying every day.

When we got home, we had to review all of the appointments I would be going to in the next few days. I would be very busy, and we hoped to find out what was causing all of my pain. When we got home, I lay down right away. I didn't feel good at all. I had a headache again, along with my neck and back pain. I wondered if I would ever find out what was wrong with me. The pain gradually began to get worse in my neck. I still had pain in my back, but my neck began to hurt more. Along with the pain in my neck, I was getting more headaches. I knew that there was something wrong, but no one else did. I couldn't help but wonder if I was going to have to live the rest of my life like this.

That night was very painful for me with awful headaches and neck pain. I could move in certain positions on the couch in order to reduce my back pain a little. However, with my neck, I couldn't find any position to help it feel better. I had something to eat and then laid down for the rest of the night and watched TV with Connie. With my moaning, I knew that Connie could not concentrate on the program she was watching. I told Connie that I needed stronger pain medication, because what I had was no longer doing the job. She told me she would call the doctor the next day. After a short time, I fell asleep, but before Connie went to bed, I had to get up a couple of times to go to the bathroom.

I was up about two times during the night, as I couldn't sleep because of the pain in my neck. I finally got to sleep and then woke up about eight o'clock the following morning. I put my clothes on and went outside and walked around. I did this, as I didn't want to wake Connie up, as my neck pain became very bad when I stood up. I immediately took a pain pill, but I began a type of moaning due to the pain, and I had to get outside. After about an hour, the pain pill helped but not enough. I went back into the house and stayed in the kitchen until I let a cupboard door go and it went crashing shut. If Connie wasn't up, she would be after that.

I waited about fifteen minutes in the kitchen, not making another sound. I figured that if I'd woken Connie up, she would be out in the kitchen fairly quickly, but she wasn't. I decided to lie down on the couch and turned on the TV to watch. I watched TV for a couple of hours, not feeling well at all, when Connie came walking into the living room. She asked how I was, and I told her. She said as soon as she washed her face, she would call the doctor's office about picking up a new prescription for pain.

She went into the bedroom, while I continued to watch TV. A short time later, she came out, picked the phone up, and made the call to the doctor. He was not in the office that morning but would be in later in the afternoon. Connie had left a message for him to call back. My pain was really getting very bad in my neck. The pain in my back had become very tolerable, but my neck was killing me. Finally, at about two o'clock, the doctor's office called and told Connie that a prescription was ready to be picked up. When Connie got dressed, we drove into Batavia to get the prescription. After picking it up, we took the prescription to the pharmacy to be filled while we waited. I hurriedly took a pill and hoped that it would give me more relief soon.

CHAPTER 3

The morning after I began taking the new pain medication, I was scheduled for a physical therapy session was at ten o'clock. I hoped that I could get through the therapy and that it would help me. I slept fairly well the previous night. The new pain pills were helping me much more, and I felt more relaxed. I hoped that the neck pain wouldn't come back worse.

It was eight o'clock in the morning, and I had to get going to get to therapy. I took a quick shower and cleaned my beard up. Since I'd been hurt, I made a pact with myself that I would not shave my beard off until I went back to work. I still had my beard but hoped it would come off soon.

After I got cleaned up, I had a piece of toast for breakfast. I could feel my neck starting to really bother me, so I took a pain pill and hoped it would help again as it did the previous night. Connie was still sleeping, and I didn't want to wake her because she was so tired. Connie had developed fibromyalgia about twelve years earlier and really suffered with pain at times. Her pain was in her muscles, and I could tell that it could be quite painful. I knew that I wouldn't like pain like that, as I would go nuts. I hoped that she would be able to sleep until noon.

My mom called me that morning to see how I was—what a woman at ninety-two years old.

After I was ready, I got in the car and drove about five minutes to my appointment. I got out of the car and noticed that I felt better than when I'd woken up. My neck still hurt but not as bad as it had been. I didn't have a headache either, so maybe I was going to have a good day. When I got inside, I had to sign in, and then I took my coat off and hung it up. I began walking around until the gentleman I had to see came to get me. It was about five minutes later when the physical therapist came out to get me. We both introduced ourselves and then went into a room with a couple of chairs and a table where I could lie down.

The physical therapist had a clipboard full of papers, and he explained that we would discuss what therapy I would be given each day. He also asked about the severity and location of the pain I was having. We talked about medication I was on and even my insurance carrier. As I expected, he was very nice, and he also happened to be the owner of the business. I explained to him what had happened and admitted that I was surprised my doctor wanted me to come to therapy. He explained that in many instances, therapy will loosen up any nerve problems a patient may have. He told me it doesn't work all of the time but also said that he'd had great success in many cases.

We completed our get-together. I would begin therapy the following Tuesday and continue seeing him every Tuesday and Thursday for a one-hour session. Before leaving, he showed me some of the machines I would be using. After the tour of the equipment, I put my coat on and left. I decided to take a ride to the local hardware store to say hello to a good friend of mine who was a part owner. I used to see him every weekend for coffee. It had been more than a month since I'd been to visit, and I felt good enough now to stop for a short time.

Seeing friends always gave me a lift. I knew that I would not be out at this store as much as I normally had been, but I needed to get out. When I pulled into the parking lot, I could tell they were kind of slow because there were not many cars there. I walked inside and said hello to everyone inside. They were all very cordial to me and asked how I was doing. They didn't know a lot about my accident and began asking me a lot of questions. I didn't mind talking about it and told them all I could. They asked if I was going back to work, and I told them that I had hoped to but didn't know when based on the pain I was having.

After spending about forty-five minutes there, I told my friends I would see them at some later date and left. I pulled into the driveway at home and went into the house. It was now about twelve thirty, and Connie was up. We gave each other a kiss, and she told me that the doctor was coming to the house at about three o'clock to talk with me. I was really glad he was coming, as I really had been very worried about many things. I was depressed to an extent. I definitely had to talk to him to get things off of my chest.

I was also glad that Connie was going to be there, because there had been some times when I hollered at her with no real reason at all. I could see that we were going to have problems that were related to the pain I was having. I became very worried that I was not going to be able to do anything around the house like I had in the past. I was worried because no one had found anything wrong with my neck of back. If there was truly nothing wrong and I continued to have so much pain, then that meant I would have to live with the pain for the rest of my life. That was going to just about kill me. I enjoyed working around the house so much, and I had my workshop that was heated for the winter and a TV and everything to work out there for hours at a time. This had really made me very depressed, and I didn't know what to do. I hoped that Dr. L could help me with my feelings.

I was starting to have more pain in my neck. It was time for me to take another pain pill, and I really hoped that this new medication would continue to take care of the pain I was having. I decided to lie down for an hour or so and have a little rest before Dr. L came. I had been lying down for an hour when Connie had to wake me up. My neck really hurt, and I didn't know why unless I had slept on it wrong. It was really bothering me and much more than it had after I'd taken a pill earlier that morning. I was going to wait for an hour or so to see if things got any better as I hoped that they would. Fortunately, the pill helped the pain in time for our meeting with Dr. L.

At three o'clock, the doorbell rang, and I went to answer it. It was Dr. L, right on time, and I was glad to see him. We shook hands, as we hadn't seen each other in a while. Connie then walked into the room and gave him a small hug and said hello. We sat down in the living room and began our mental therapy session. He had to be brought up to date about my accident. He was very surprised to hear of the circumstance in which I fell down the stairs and was surprised that I was not hurt worse than I was. I explained all of the things that had been going through my mind, including worrying about my pay and Connie losing her job.

When I told him about my thoughts of suing the people involved, he told me that I needed to put things in perspective, as I was trying to deal with too many things at once. The comments pertained to me putting the problems that I had in order of importance. He felt that we were definitely dealing with a lot of negative situations, but he felt we would get through it by dealing with everything one day at a time. We talked for another fifteen minutes, and our hour was up. I felt quite better mentally when we were done, but my neck began to hurt quite a bit.

Dr. L left, and I was so happy, as I really had to lie down due to my neck. I hadn't felt much pain in my back for the past few days. I didn't know why, but I was glad I didn't have to deal with the same pain from both my neck and back at the same time. I went to lie down for a while and fell asleep for a short time. When I woke up, Connie reminded me that we must go into Rochester the following day to get the MRI for our next appointment in Batavia. It was November 7, 2000, and I decided to have Connie call the doctor again to get stronger medicine for my neck. The pain was really getting out of hand, and I couldn't continue like this. I figured my doctor must think I was a real pain in the ass, but the pain was unbelievable, as it continued to increase at will.

Before my back and neck injury, I'd never had any pain that continually increased. In fact, it had always been just the opposite with the pain decreasing as I felt better. I found myself becoming very confused, as there were things happening to me that had become quite different than before that damn fall. I can remember thinking, *I hope that there aren't too many more unique things happening to me.*

Connie made the phone call to the neurologist's office and left word for him to call her. She had told the receptionist that I needed stronger pain medication, as I was having quite a bit more pain. We hoped he would call back fairly soon so we could pick the new prescription up before we had to go to Rochester for the new tests. About an hour later, the phone rang, and it was the doctor. He and Connie talked for about five minutes, and she was answering questions about my pain. Connie told him that the pain had increased quite a bit in the past couple of days. The doctor agreed to write a new prescription, which would be ready in an hour.

Connie had to go in and clean up a little bit before she was ready to leave. I didn't feel good at all, but I told her I would ride with her to get the prescription. We left in about forty minutes. I would run in to get the prescription from the doctor's office, so we could drive back to Le Roy and go right to the pharmacy. When we got there, I ran into the office and got the prescription. We drove right back to Le Roy, and I took the prescription right to the pharmacy. I had to wait about twenty minutes. Connie had come in to walk around and just look in general. I knew that if she came in that we would be buying something, and she did. The prescription was done in about thirty minutes, and we left. As soon as we got home, I took a pill and lay down.

After discovering a few weeks earlier what had happened to my insides, including the trouble I was having urinating, I was very worried about what I'd done to the inside of my body when I fell down those damn stairs. I realized I must have seriously hurt something to have this happen. I wished that I knew what it was and hoped that the x-rays or MRI would tell. At least, I sure hoped they would. My concern was that if these two things had cropped up, was it possible that I could have damaged something else worse?

It seemed as though I may have hurt a nerve somewhere in my back that controlled how and when I went to the bathroom. Although that possibility really scared me, I realized there was nothing I could do about it at the moment. I knew that I would have to wait to see if we could find something out about my problems.

I went back to see my neurologist later that afternoon. I thanked him for giving me the stronger pills and explained how the pain in my neck was increasing at such a very fast pace, although I didn't know why. He had hoped to see something in the films we brought him to reevaluate. He began looking at them and didn't notice anything out of the ordinary.

He decided to send me to an anesthesiologist who could inject cortisone shots into my neck. He was hopeful that the shots would loosen up my neck in all the places where I was experiencing the pain. But before I went to the anesthesiologist, he wanted me to see a neurosurgeon in Rochester. He also ordered a new MRI, which I would take with me to the appointment. I agreed that this course of action sounded like the right thing to do in order to hopefully find out what the problem may be. We ended the meeting with a prescription to the anesthesiologist.

Connie and I left his office and decided to stop and have some lunch at a local diner. I didn't know how it was going to turn out, as I hadn't sat down in a long time. When I sat down in our booth, it didn't feel too bad, but I knew I'd have to wait and see how it felt in thirty minutes. After fifteen minutes passed, I was up and had to walk around, because my back was bothering me. I walked for a short time and then sat down again. I sat for about ten minutes and had to get up again. I realized I wouldn't be able to sit for much time at all. After we were served our meals, I rushed to eat mine as fast as I could. I normally didn't like rushing, but I was afraid I would be up and down many times before I finished my lunch. That was our first time out to eat since I'd been hurt, and I didn't think it went too bad.

I think that Connie enjoyed that we stopped to eat, but I know she didn't like me getting up as much as I did. But, she knew my problem and didn't complain at all. When we arrived home, I decided to lie down. I was pretty tired and needed to rest awhile. Connie rested as well, as we had to get up at eight o'clock the next morning for our appointment with the neurologist at ten thirty.

It was now one thirty on the afternoon of November 9, and we were both very tired. I was especially tired because of our meal out. Although I had, indeed, I made it through, I was still in pain. This time, it was my back. My neck was still the major problem, but trying to sit down to eat was really a challenge. It was good to be home where we could relax.

Connie had to call the neurosurgeon's office in Rochester to set up an appointment with him. But before we could see him, I had to have another MRI. After Connie had called the doctor's office, she called Borg Imaging to set up an appointment for the new MRI. Connie got the neurosurgeon's office on the phone and made the appointment for November 18, 2000, at three o'clock in Rochester. She then called Borg Imaging and scheduled the appointment for the MRI to be done on November 16, 2000.

CHAPTER 4

Why did this whole thing happen to me? What did I do to deserve all of this? I have been told that there is a reason for everything, but why me? What could I have done to deserve living like this? These questions ran through my head, but I knew that I had to quit feeling sorry for myself. It happened, and there was nothing I could do to change that. I realized that so many other people in this world were much worse off than I was, and they didn't do anything to deserve it. To this day, I get very upset when I see all of the children with cancer. They may not make it through all of the rough times they face. These are the children who have it rough, not me.

Finally, the day arrived when I would go to get my MRI for the neurosurgeon. I had been through the MRI before and really didn't care for it all. However, I realized that it was necessary if we were going to get to the bottom of all of my pain.

On that day, my neck was really painful, but the pills seemed to help quite a bit. Connie and I drove to Rochester, and I got out of the car very stiff and in a lot of pain. I walked around for a few minutes to straighten up as much as I could. We walked inside, and I signed in. We were told to sit down and relax for a few minutes. I began to walk around when a lady appeared in the doorway and called my name. I went with her through the door to another very large room with the MRI machine in it.

In front of me was a very hard table that I would have to lie on. It was the kind of surface that created so much pain in my back by lying on it. I held my breath and sat on the table as best I could and then swung my legs around to place them on the table. The procedure took about an hour, and my pain was very bad. My back really hurt, but I couldn't take a pain pill for another hour and a half. What else was new?

Connie and I left and would pick the films up before seeing the neurosurgeon in a couple of days. We had been doing so much running around, and I knew that it had become very hard on Connie. Having to do all of this and working had to be very tough on her. I told her I would find someone else to help us out by taking me to appointments, but she wanted to be there. On top of everything else, I couldn't help but think about the fact that Connie would not have a job after February. We had no choice but to deal with everything when it was time. It was so nice that the doctors she worked for allow her to cart me around to have all these tests and go to so many appointments.

After we arrived home, I lay down with a lot of pain, but at least I was able to take another pain pill in a matter of minutes.

The pain from both my neck and back was indescribable. Unless you have dealt with the same pain, it's impossible to even imagine how bad the pain was. Only then would someone know what true pain is.

I lay down for a couple of hours, and then I got up and walked around for a few minutes. Connie had to go back to work, so I was home alone the rest of the day until she came home for the night. I didn't do much at all for the rest of the day. I guess that I lay down most of the time, as there wasn't anything else I could do. At about five o'clock, Connie walked through the door, and I asked how her day went. She told me that it wasn't too bad, but they were quite busy when she got back to work from our appointments. Connie sat down and had a cup of coffee, and I didn't feel too bad. I asked her if I could order a pizza for dinner, and she thought the idea was great, as she was too tired to cook. I ordered the pizza and we eventually got it and ate it. I stayed up lying on the couch for a few hours and then kissed Connie good night and eventually fell asleep. My back and neck were not too bad, as I had taken another pain pill about an hour earlier.

I woke up the next morning and remembered that I didn't have any appointments that day. My exercise sessions had stopped a week earlier because I had so many other appointments scheduled and because I was so tired. Connie went to work at seven thirty and kissed me good-bye before she left. The day went by fairly quickly because I slept most of the day. I had been very tired from the MRI the day before and needed these days in between appointments to relax.

My next appointment was the following day, and I was hopeful that it would be the day of truth. I was really praying that I would find out from the neurosurgeon what was wrong with me after he looked at the films we would bring with us. We would soon get some answers—I hoped.

After Connie returned home from work, the rest of the day was quiet. She sat on the love seat to read the paper and fell asleep. We didn't eat until about eight thirty that night, which was all right with me as she had worked hard all day. The next day was Saturday, and we still had to leave for an appointment. I hoped she'd be able to sleep on Sunday.

On Saturday, I was up at about eight o'clock. Because I'd gotten so much sleep the day before, I was up several times during the night. I would watch TV at times and then listen to the radio, but I made it through the night with a little sleep anyway. I woke Connie up at about ten o'clock, so she would have time to relax awhile before we had to shower and do all the things we had to do before leaving. I had not felt too bad because all of the pills I was able to take without doing much to create a lot of pain.

Finally, at one o'clock, we got into the car and were off to pick up the films from my recent MRI. After getting them, we drove to Strong Hospital for our meeting with the neurosurgeon. We arrived a little early, so I walked around while Connie sat down in a chair with a magazine. After about fifteen minutes, the neurosurgeon came in and introduced himself, and we did the same. Connie handed the MRI results to him, and he looked at the film for about five minutes. He then told us that he wanted me to have a CAT scan and myelogram. He also said that he wanted me to have another MRI because there was a question in the film we had just given him and he wanted to see another MRI from a different provider. He also explained that he might recommend going ahead with cortisone shots in my neck, but he would decide after his review of the new films.

When we left the doctor's office, I was not happy at all. We really didn't find out any information that we didn't already know. It was depressing, as I had seen so many different professional people and still didn't know any more than I did the day after I fell down the stairs. I was upsetting to not know why I was experiencing so much pain. I tried to keep a very positive attitude about everything, but at that point, I hadn't been able to. I had to keep remembering the small kids I saw at St. Jude Children's Research Hospital to realize how fortunate I was to even be alive. Many of those poor little children wouldn't even be alive in another year. I hoped that if I ever felt better, I would somehow be able to help other people less fortunate.

We arrived home after the visit with the neurosurgeon. I really didn't know what was going to happen to me next, but I imagined I would find out from someone fairly soon. I knew that I would have to start therapy again. I really didn't even get started with therapy yet, but I decided I'd better call and get my dates set up. When I got into the house, I lay down. My pain was quite intense, but I wanted to wait as long as I could until I couldn't stand it anymore before I took the medication. I feared I would be so drugged up that I would never get off of the drugs. My mother always told us kids to stay away from any kind of drugs. I realized my situation was very different, but I still had those awful pills going into my system.

Ten minutes after thinking about really holding off before taking the medication, I had to go into the kitchen to take a pain pill. The pain became so great that I had to take it—and right away. How stupid was I? Those damn pills were keeping my sanity, whatever sanity I had left. I lay down again and must have dozed off for a while, as I heard Connie come in the back door. When we got home, she wanted to go uptown to get a few things. That was about an hour and a half earlier. She had picked some things up to eat for dinner.

After we ate dinner, I decided to go through some old papers. I began to set a file up to keep things in better order. My life had been almost at a standstill regarding trying to do anything other than lying down or walking around. So, I found a pillow that was pretty comfortable and sat on the couch to go through all of the old papers we had in the cupboard. It was the place we put our checkbook, current bills that had to be paid during the month, and copies of the bills that had already been paid. I had to have something to do that would be beneficial to the house. I had to feel that I was really doing something around the house.

It took me about two hours to set up a system to organize the bills paid and the bills to be paid. This had not been done in almost a year. Due to my laziness and my injury, I just never did anything. When I was all done, it was time to take a pain pill. I had noticed during the past couple of days that my neck was beginning to hurt quite a bit more. I didn't know how long it was going to be before I had to ask my doctor for stronger pain pills again, but I knew what I was taking at the time was really strong.

I keep telling myself and Connie that something very bad had happened to my neck. I often found myself thinking back to the time when I fell. I went head over heels after I slipped on the glue that had been put on the steel and concrete stairs. When I stopped sliding, my neck hit a step very hard, and I was knocked out for a period of time. Every professional I had seen me said the same thing—nothing could be found in x-rays or any of the other tests that had been done to and around my head.

I finished my filing and decided to lie down and watch TV before going to bed. Connie watched with me. When the show ended at eleven, it was time for me to go to bed. Connie was going to stay up for a while longer. I lay on the couch and coasted off to sleep. I had woken up two or three times during the night to go to the bathroom. I eventually woke up at eight o'clock and made some breakfast for myself. It was Saturday, so Connie was going to sleep in. She really needed some sleep, as she was always worried about me. She should have been worrying about herself more.

Connie and I had been married almost thirty-five years, and since 1986 , she had dealt with a medical problem called fibromyalgia, which is also a form of chronic pain. She lived in pain every single day of her life. Muscle pain, back pain, headaches, neck pain, and depression all created her own type of hell that she had to deal with while taking care of me. She very seldom complained, but when she did, I could only surmise how bad she felt. She was the only one who truly knew what she was going through. With my condition, she had to also take on making sure that I got to doctors' appointments and anything else regarding the pain I was experiencing. She deserved so much for all she went through.

It is now November of 2000 and things aren't any better for me. I decided that if I ever got better, I would grant her anything she wanted within the realm of us being able to afford it. I wished that we had more money so I could have hired a maid or some other type of assistant to take me, and even Connie, to appointments.

CHAPTER 5

On December 4th of 2000 I decided that I'd like to take Connie to an early dinner in Batavia if she would like to go. I didn't know how I would feel when it was time to leave, but I could try. I thought that she would appreciate if we could go out to eat.

Connie woke up at about ten o'clock that morning and thanked me for letting her sleep. Of course, she never had to thank me, because I knew that she needed the rest. If it were up to me, she would have it. After about an hour or so, I asked her if she would like to go for an early dinner in Batavia. She told me that she wasn't sure if she wanted to go but would let me know a little later. I told her that was fine.

About forty-five minutes later, I needed to take a pain pill. I was starting to get an awful headache. I never used to get headaches, but since falling down the stairs, I seemed to get them quite a bit. Although I didn't get migraines, they were still are very painful. I decided to lie down for a while to see if it went away. About an hour later, Connie came into the living room and said she would like to go to dinner if I still wanted to go. I told her whenever she could get ready, we would go. She asked if we could go at three thirty. I agreed that the time was fine.

At about one thirty, Connie began to get ready to go to dinner. I was kind of looking forward to this, as it would only be my second time out. My neck was hurting quite a bit, and I began to worry that the pain would be so great that I'd have to back out. The way I had it figured, I would be able to take a pain pill at about three, which would be the perfect time for the medication to get into my blood stream and give me an hour of feeling pretty good for our dinner out. At three o'clock, I took the pill, and Connie was also ready. I had to take a quick shower, which would make me feel even better. Soon, we were ready to go and on our way to Batavia.

There was one restaurant in town I liked, because it had booths and the cushions were fairly comfortable. I also brought a pillow from home to sit on. On the way to the restaurant, I thought perhaps it was time to order a special pillow to use whenever I had to sit down. When we arrived at the diner, we were happy to find a booth still available. We went to sit down, and I sat on the pillow I'd brought along.

The waitress immediately came to our table with glasses of water and two menus. I began to feel my pain pill cutting in and making me feel better. I was very concerned about me sitting down for so long, as I knew I would pay for it later. I always enjoyed taking Connie out to eat if she wasn't in a lot of pain.

We decided on the food and gave the waitress our order. About ten minutes had gone by since we'd arrived, and I had to get up to walk a little. Connie knew I had to do this, so she just said okay. I walked to the bathroom just to loosen up and then went back to the table and sat down. Soon after, the meals were brought to our table, and we began to eat. I had gotten through about half of my meal when I had to get up again to walk. I knew that people would begin looking at me making my second trip to the restroom in such a short time. I didn't care, though, because I knew how bad the pain would be if I didn't get up to walk. When I got back to the table, I finished my meal. Connie was still eating, and I hoped she would finish before I had to get up to walk again. Connie knew that I was anxious and said she would hurry so we could leave. I assured her that she could take her time. She finally finished about five minutes later, and we paid the bill and left.

As I began to get into the car, I realized that I had left my pillow in the restaurant, so I had to go back in to get it. We were finally ready to head back home to Le Roy. About twenty minutes later, we pulled into the garage. I got out of the car and had to walk around for a while. Connie had gotten her key and went into the house. After walking for about ten or fifteen minutes, I went into the house. Connie hugged and kissed me and thanked me for taking her out. I knew that it wouldn't happen again for quite some time, but at least I made her happy for the moment.

Thinking about the pillow for my butt at the restaurant, I started looking for a good pillow once we got back home. I found one that looked like it would really help me. It had a round opening in the back, so my spine and butt would be free from any pressure. I showed it to Connie before I ordered it to get her input. She looked at it and agreed that it would help me when I had to sit down. The pillow was about fifty dollars and was made out of fairly hard foam. I did some research online about the compression by weight for the density of foam in the pillow and was able to get what I felt would really help me. I placed the order, which was supposed to arrive in about a week.

After placing the order, I realized that my neck had begun to hurt quite a bit. I knew that after going out to dinner and having to sit as long as I did, I was bound to be in pain. I would get over it, but I had to suffer in the meantime. My goal was to make my beautiful wife happy.

I knew that on Monday I was going to have to get in touch with my neurologist to get some stronger medication. I was sure he would go crazy when I came back yet again for an increase in medication. At that time, Connie had felt fairly good for the past day or so. I hoped that I don't have to start traveling again and putting pressure on her to get me to appointments.

I finally had to lie down and relax. My neck was quite painful, but it let up a little when my head hit the pillow. I was very tired, as was Connie. I decided to take a small nap and was sure that she would do the same. The whole experience had really been very tiresome, and I still hadn't found anyone to tell me what the hell was wrong with my neck and back. When I really stopped to think about it, there were times when I wasn't sure if I really wanted to know what was wrong with me. I feared it may scare the hell out of me.

Since we'd already had our dinner, after resting for a couple of hours, we planned on watching some TV together. About an hour before our shows started, I thought that I heard a noise in Connie's bedroom, so I knew I wouldn't have to try and wake her up. She appeared about ten minutes later and asked how I felt. I told her I was feeling pretty good and then asked her how she felt. She said that she was okay.

Just before the program came on TV, the phone rang; it was my sister. She wanted to know how things were and apologized for not having called sooner. I told her that all was pretty good at the moment but then asked if it would be possible to call her the following day, as Connie and I were getting ready to watch a good program on TV. We agreed to speak the following day.

Connie and I began watching the movie together, and she watched it to the end. Unfortunately, I fell asleep about an hour into the movie. As Connie began closing blinds and turning lights off for the night, I woke up and noticed it was time to go to bed. I was on my bed, but she was walking down the hall to her bedroom. It was too late to say anything, and I didn't want to scare her. She went into her room and closed the door. I normally liked to kiss her good night, but it was a time that I didn't make it in time. I had gone into my room to put on my pajamas, took a pill, and went to bed. I lay down on the couch and went to sleep—hopefully for the night.

I woke up Sunday morning without having to get up during the night. Then I had to go to the bathroom, as I was filled to the top. I immediately had to take a pain pill for the pain in my neck. All I could think of was calling the neurologist first thing Monday to get stronger medicine. At this point in time, I started to become very depressed. I had tried to handle everything the best I could, but I realized that I was starting to come apart. I was feeling funny inside and getting very sweaty, and I didn't know why. I felt so lousy but couldn't explain what the feeling was. I had never felt that way before. I prayed to God that it would go away, as I was very nervous and didn't know what to do. I can remember hoping the feeling would go away before Connie woke up, because I didn't want to worry her.

After an hour or so, the feelings I had inside started to go away. Again, I thanked God for helping me out. Connie didn't need any more problems. At about eleven o'clock, Connie came walking into the living room. I was lying on the couch and feeling okay again. She asked me how things were, and I told her okay. The truth was the pain in my neck was beginning to get worse, and I was going crazy with my rollercoaster ride of pain. I decided to make the call to my doctor the next morning.

I woke up at about seven o'clock on the morning of Monday, December 4, 2000. I had to take a pain pill right away because of the pain. Either Connie or I needed to call the doctor. I also had to call the neurosurgeon about the cortisone shots he wanted me to have. I didn't know anything more than he wanted me to try the shots before anything else was done.

At nine o'clock, Connie called my neurologist's office and requested a call back from the doctor to discuss the pain medication. After Connie made that call, she called the neurosurgeon to find out about the cortisone shots for my neck. She also left word for him to call me back.

I decided to have some breakfast and was hoping that I would hear from both doctors soon. The first call came through at about eleven thirty from the neurologist. Connie had picked up the phone and told him that my pain had increased a lot in the past couple of weeks. She told him that we'd seen the neurosurgeon, and the only thing he'd mentioned was for me to have cortisone shots. The doctor said that he would write a new prescription, and we could pick it up in the afternoon. I was very happy to hear that, but the neurosurgeon did not call back that day. We left the answering service on when we drove to Batavia to get the prescription but didn't receive any calls.

We picked the prescription up, and I was relieved to be able to make it through the day without all of the pain. My pain level consistently ran between a six and an eight with the new pills. After my accident, my pain was initially at about a four but had gradually increased to an eight.

By December 31, 2000, I continued to wonder why the pain kept increasing in my neck. I'd had MRIs, CAT scans, myleograms, and x-rays with nothing showing on anything. I was beginning to wonder if it was time to find other doctors. At this point, I'd had three different doctors, and no one had discovered what my problems were.

At times, I thought that maybe there was nothing wrong with me, and it was all in my head. I couldn't believe that was the case, but I also couldn't understand why no one had found any problems with my neck. Supposedly, the doctors whom I had seen were very good at what they do. Everything that was going on had affected me badly. Mentally, I didn't know what to think or what to do to get through all of this without going to pieces.

I can remember thinking, *What if this is all a dream, and there is nothing really wrong with me?* I hoped that I didn't have a mental breakdown, as I was feeling very funny inside of my body. It was something I'd never felt before. I didn't know what I was going to do but hoped to figure it out with the help of all of the nurses in our family. Fortunately my wife, daughter and sister are all nurses and I am sure that one of them could find the answer for me.

I continually prayed to my God to help me through this entire nightmare. *Why did this happen to me, and what did I do to deserve it?* I wondered. I knew that there were people who had it much worse off than I did, but the continued pain was really driving me nuts. I hoped that God heard my prayers, as it was becoming tougher and tougher to get through this.

CHAPTER 6

On December 7, 2000, I began with my cortisone shots. I had to have a shot once a week, and the doctor was hoping that I would get some relief from them. The first shot I had felt exceptionally good and cut my pain a lot. I hadn't felt so good in a long time. At the time, I thought that if I felt that good after each shot, I would be in good shape.

Unfortunately, the effect of the shot wore off later on in the day, and I was right back to being in a lot of pain again. This was not good, as I felt like I'd received false hope of feeling better. Once again, I found myself wondering if this was what I would have to go through each week. I was right back on my strong medication for the pain, as my body realized the shot provided just a short period of relief. I realized I'd just have to see what happened the following week.

I had gone back to see the anesthesiologist for six different visits, which turned out to be nothing but a big bomb. Each session was the same as the first. I would feel good for a few hours after the injection, and then I was back to the pain and all. Needless to say, I probably should have stopped with the shots after the second when we realized they would not help me. I know that a lot of money could have been saved.

I was going to begin seeing my new pain specialist. He was from Buffalo and had just stared a new practice in Batavia one day a week. He was affiliated with Sports Medicine in Batavia. Dr. L had given him a good recommendation, so we decided to see how good he was. I really needed someone to help me with my drugs when my pain got out of control. It hadn't been bad the past week or so. The last prescription I received from the neurologist seemed to be helping me get through each day.

My first meeting with Dr. B was on January 16, 2001, at his office in Batavia. He wanted me to have an MRI before my first visit. Connie and I went to Borg Imaging in Rochester to have an MRI done, which made my fifth MRI since being hurt four months earlier.

We arrived at Dr. B's office, and I was a little nervous. I guess the reason was that I was desperately trying to find a doctor who could help me with anything. I had yet to find a doctor who could have empathy for me. The past four months had been awful, and I hadn't found anyone who could really understand what I was dealing with.

Dr. B was kind of a tough doctor who spoke very deeply. I could tell that he had the knowledge in the profession in which he practiced. We talked for a short period of time while he reviewed the results from my latest MRI.

He allowed me to continue on the same drug that had been prescribed for me a couple of weeks earlier but mentioned he would probably make some changes at our next visit. Our appointments were set up for every Monday. I had just finished with the doctor who was shooting me full of cortisone, and it was great to not have to see him anymore. As the next few days went by, I again began to have an increase in my neck pain. This really bothered me, as I'd never heard anyone else whose pain kept escalating over a period of four weeks. I found comfort in the fact that I'd be seeing Dr. B again soon. I was sure he would take care of my problem.

We had an appointment at one o'clock on Monday, and I was all set to tell him about the pain I had in my neck. When we got to his office, I mentioned the increase in pain when he asked how I was. It was then that the doctor mentioned he was going to put me on a fentanyl patch. He felt that I would feel less pain going on the patch beginning. He started me at a dose of twenty-five micrograms. It really looked like at least my pain specialist had been up to speed on how I felt. All I cared about was that the patches kept my pain under control so I wouldn't suffer like I had in the past on the pills.

With the new fentanyl patch, things were a little different at first. Instead of putting tablets down my throat, I was putting this patch on my arm, and I had to remember to change it every third day. It would take a little time to get used to this, but I knew I would be able to adjust. The patch helped me more than all of the pills I'd been taking.

The pain seemed to be better for a short time, but then my neck really began to hurt an awful lot again. My doctor increased the strength of my patch during the next six months to one hundred micrograms, which helped me a lot. However, I was very concerned about becoming addicted to the patch. The doctor assured me that as long as the medication was controlling my pain, I didn't need to worry. The fentanyl patch is supposedly one hundred times stronger than morphine. One of the problems I had run into with my pharmacy was that they could not get the patch at times, which meant I had to go to other pharmacies to get it. Connie and I saw where this could become a big problem in the future. Fortunately, it only happened a couple of times.

A couple of weeks went by, and I had a Monday appointment with Dr. B. I hadn't been feeling good that day and was kind of nervous and worried about things that I couldn't put my finger on. I'd felt the same way once before. I was worried about things I wasn't even sure of.

The receptionist showed Connie and me to the examining room and closed the door. As I sat in the room, I finally had a cold sweat and really felt very funny inside almost like things were caving in on me. I began to wonder if I was having a nervous breakdown.

The doctor came into the room and greeted us. Connie looked at me and asked me if there was something wrong. I kind of looked back at her in a daze, and then it happened. I began crying uncontrollably and shaking all over. This lasted for about five to ten minutes. When I calmed down, the doctor told us that I had to see a psychiatrist as soon as possible. He told me that I'd just had a panic attack. Connie explained that we had been looking and hoped to find one soon. After a short conversation, we left.

When we got into the car, Connie asked how I felt. I told her that I had calmed down, but I didn't know what had come over me. I just wasn't sure. Connie made no comments, and then we were on our way home. When we got home, I went inside to lie down for a while. Connie came in and began looking for Dr. L's phone number. She was going to call again to see if there were any openings for a new patient.

Unfortunately, she was told that there were still no openings, but the receptionist said they would call when one was available. Connie had told me of the problem and mentioned that we had to see someone. We didn't want to go to Rochester, so she began looking in the Batavia phone book. After coming up with a name and number, she placed a call. The new office did, indeed, have openings, so Connie booked an appointment for the following week for me to see the doctor.

Connie's last day at work was going to be February 28, 2001. I knew that she was bothered by this, but I definitely needed her home with me. We had investments to help us make it through financially until I got on disability. Unfortunately, I didn't know when that would happen. I was receiving workman's compensation and had a disability insurance policy that I'd paid on through work for many years. When I received payments from the policy, we would be all set for a while. I told Connie not to worry, but I realized that was easier said than done.

I still had been feeling funny inside. I couldn't help but wonder why I'd had that damn panic attack asI figured that I must be really worrying about something. I realized that with all the drugs I was on, I had acquired an I-don't-give-a-shit attitude. At least the pain was not as bad as it has been, but the time had come to tell my doctor that the pain was getting worse again.

One particular Friday I found myself experiencing that same funny feeling that I'd had at the doctor's office. I decided to spend much of the morning lying down. Jen was stopping over in a few hours to hang out with us. We hadn't seen her in a few days. I hoped that I would be okay.

About ten o'clock that morning, Jenny showed up, and I was really feeling worse. I remember wishing that I know what I could do to shake this awful feeling. I went into my bedroom and prayed to God that this feeling would go away. After a few minutes, I came out of the bedroom.

I lay down on the couch, and then it happened. I completely went to pieces. I began crying uncontrollably and was told later that I was saying things that evidently were not making any sense. After Connie and Jenny talked about the problem, they decided that the best thing would be to take me to the hospital. And so, Connie called for the ambulance, which came in about twenty minutes. The ambulance crew came into the house and loaded me on to the gurney. It appeared that I had more problems that I was worried about than I realized. I was put in the ambulance, and we headed for Strong in Rochester. We arrived about thirty minutes later, and I was wheeled into the emergency room where I was given a shot to calm me down.

After being reevaluated by a doctor, I was taken to the floor where they treated people with emotional problems. When I got to my room, a nurse was there to perform all the necessary tests. Connie and Jen had followed the ambulance by car. They came to the room and talked with the doctor, who had just arrived. After a few minutes, they came into my room. They told me I was going to have to spend some time there to get straightened out.

The days were slow, but I knew that I had to clear my head of all the things that were bothering me. I had been really worried about all that was happening and didn't really let it sink in. After a week, I was ready to go home. Connie came to pick me up, and we were on the way. We began talking about what had happened, and Connie mentioned that I definitely needed to see a psychiatrist as soon as possible. Fortunately, Connie had made an appointment for the following week. When we got home, I went right to the couch.

The phone began to ring as if everyone knew I was home. It was Jen on the phone, and she sent her love. I then gave the phone to Connie. As I lay there, my neck began to hurt quite a bit. I had been changing the patches as required, but they didn't seem to take care of the problem. I decided that I would talk to Dr. B when I saw him. I must have dozed off for an hour or so, but the phone rang and woke me up. It was a friend who wanted to tell me that he was glad I was home and was willing to help around the house if needed.

The day had come for my meeting with the new psychiatrist, and we were finally on the way to see him. I was hopeful that he'd be good and would be able to help me out. After signing in at his office, Connie sat down, and I paced.

Finally, he walked into the waiting area and showed us into his office. I could tell right away that I did not care for him. He began talking and asking me questions. When he asked me, "What do you think it will take to straighten you out?" I made up my mind that I wouldn't be back. I was relieved when it was time to head for home. I had depression, but he won't be my doctor.

As we were driving, I told Connie I could not go back to him again, and she totally agreed. We arrived at home about twenty minutes later and went into the house. Connie knew that we had to find another doctor and began looking through the phone book while I lay down. After a few minutes, she found the name of a different doctor in Batavia. This doctor worked for the State of New York. Connie wrote the name down and planned to call at another time. Connie then lay down also, as she was tired.

CHAPTER 7

On March 6, 2001, I had an appointment with Dr. B in Batavia. We arrived a little early, and the doctor had walked by us as we came in and said hello. We signed in and sat down. In about five minutes, we were called into his office.

We started out talking about my hospital stay. I explained that I was definitely being treated for depression. He told me not to be ashamed, as I had been through an awful lot in the past few months. He asked about the psychiatrist, and we told him of our experiences and explained we were still looking. I also told him that the patch didn't appear to be doing the job any longer, as my pain had begun to increase significantly. He then wrote a prescription for 100 micrograms, which he said should take care of the problem. He also told me that he wanted the new patch to be changed every other day instead of every third day. After talking about another twenty minutes, we left.

I started back up with my physical therapy sessions and began going three days a week. I agreed to do what the doctors wanted me to do, but I didn't feel like it was putting me any closer to finding out the problem with my neck and back. I decided that I would go on a regular basis until I didn't feel like going. They had me doing quite a bit during my sessions. As part of my therapy, I began with the TENS unit. This is a device that gives electrical impulses to the area that hurts. In a way, it soothed the area and felt relaxing.

I also had another appointment with Dr. L, who was the friend of mine. He had helped me a lot since I'd been seeing him. He dealt with me as a new patient and really had me open up to him. I wish that he could dispense drugs but understood that he couldn't.

The new patch was working okay, and I hoped that it would continue to do so. The rest of the day I lay around. Connie went out to get some groceries, and I watched a little TV. When Connie got home, she began to cook a new meal she'd read about in some magazine. Once again, I was the guinea pig.

We had a fairly late dinner, and after cleaning up, I was kind of tired and decided to lie down. Connie began reading the paper, and I slipped off into a light sleep. I must have slept for about an hour when the phone rang. It was our daughter calling to see how things were. Connie had told Jenny that I was doing pretty well and that she'd just returned home from shopping. Connie then got up and went to some other room to talk. I slipped off to sleep, and before I knew it, the time was one thirty in the morning, and the whole house was dark. I had to go to the bathroom but then went back to sleep.

I was up at about eight o'clock and decided to take a ride to see my friend at Ace Hardware, I went out there, made some coffee, and hung around there for about an hour before coming back home. I had an appointment with my doctor that afternoon and decided I needed to go to Batavia. I got to the doctor's office and spent an hour there talking about my depression, which had landed me in the hospital. He was really good for me.

I needed to see a psychiatrist, and Connie had found one who worked for the state. She made an appointment for a couple of days later. Those few days went by quickly. My neck began to hurt more than it had since I'd started using the new strength patch. I kept thinking that something was wrong in my head. I didn't know what it was, but I continued to have pain in my neck. The strength of the patch was very strong. Although I didn't like to take such strong drugs, the pain was just too bad if I didn't.

I had gotten used to the patch and not having all of the intense pain, so I couldn't really complain.

I had been thinking about something in the months since I'd been hurt. Someone from the place I worked came to see me once, and then I never received another visitor from work. I gave all I could to that company, and no one came to see me.

Another thing that upset me a great deal is that I should have let Connie sue them. There was no way of knowing what would happen to me during the next couple of years. I have never been out to just sue someone, but I also had to make sure that we were taken care of. I made a very bad call on that one. I really didn't take care of us like I normally did. I hoped it wouldn't bite me in the ass later.

Finally, the day came to see the new psychiatrist for the state. I hoped he was better than the last one I saw. Our appointment was at three o'clock in the afternoon, and the day flew by for some reason. When it was time to leave, we got into the car and made the short trip to Batavia. We went to this big building where all the state offices were. I asked where this gentleman was, and they directed me to another area down the hallway. .

We finally found his location and signed in. Connie sat down while I paced around. Soon, a lady came in and read my name. We then followed her to the doctor's office. When he came in, I noted that he was in his early sixties. We chatted for about an hour, and I told him all about myself. We made another appointment for the following week. He had these hard chairs in his office, and I walked during our full session.

As we were driving home, Connie asked me what I thought of him, and I told her he was okay. I still was not totally happy with him, but I needed him for my depression. Dr. B insisted that I have this doctor. We got home, and I found my usual spot on the couch. My neck had hurt a little that afternoon, but I had also taken a hydrocodone to lighten the pain. Connie told me she was going to call Dr. L's office to see if they had any openings for new patients yet.

I couldn't believe that she said great to the person on the phone. She made the appointment for two days later at two o'clock in the afternoon. I was finally going to have the psychiatrist I had been waiting to see for so long. I was so happy. Connie had told me she would call the other doctor for the state and cancel the appointment we just made.

Connie called and cancelled my appointment with the psychiatrist for the state the next day. I also had my new appointment with Dr. Le. We would meet soon, and I could really go over things that were bothering me.

My mom was ninety-two years old, and ever since my dad passed away in June 1985, I had vowed to watch out for her. My older sister, Rozella, who was the firstborn, took care of all the things in the house and took her to doctors' appointments and the like. I took care of everything outside the house. This went on until the day I fell and was hurt. From that point on, my sister had to take care of everything.

My mom was such a nice lady. She always liked to get together with her lady friends to play cards. She was also on the computer all the time, playing card games and whatever else she learned to do. She just loved it. Mom was very worried about me and was continually calling or coming by to make sure her baby boy was okay.

My sister Elaine lived in Colorado. She moved from Rochester a number of years earlier, as her husband worked for Eastman Kodak. My other sister Sharon lived in Connecticut. She'd moved there with her husband and kids also many years ago. They both come home whenever needed.

I was back to my therapy sessions, along with seeing my pain specialist and other special doctors. By this time, we had added many miles on Connie's car from having to drive all over the place. I could not believe how many doctors I had to see. And still, I knew that despite all of these doctors, no one had come up with an answer to all of the problems I had. Now that I was seeing so many doctors, I was sure that within the next twenty years they might find out what was wrong with me.

CHAPTER 8

One night I went to bed for the evening and quickly dozed off on the couch. I slept pretty well until about four o'clock in the morning when I woke up with light chest pains. I really didn't think too much of it, as I'd had these types of pains before. I was quite sure that it was indigestion, and I just needed to get rid of the gas that was irritating my system. I got up and walked around for a while, as that normally helped me. But that time, I was wrong. Instead of relieving the discomfort, the pain got stronger, and then I began to worry.

When I check the time, I saw it was five thirty. I didn't want to wake Connie up, as I knew that she really needed her sleep. I even thought about hopping in the car and driving to the emergency room myself, but I knew that Connie would be very upset with me. I decided to wait another hour or two if I could. I hoped that maybe by then I wouldn't even have to wake her up. What a stupid move that was, as the pain really got very intense. I realized I had to wake her up immediately.

I went into her room and gently shook her as I quietly told her I wasn't feeling well. She replied back asking me what the problem was. I told her that I had awful chest pains. Evidently, that was the right thing to say, as she sprung out of bed. The look on her face was one of great concern.

My neck was hurting, but gradually, the chest pains became more intense than my neck. Connie got up and immediately went to get the cuff to take my blood pressures. When she was done, she immediately went and called the ambulance. After getting off the phone, she made sure that I was as comfortable as I could be. She then went in to get dressed. When she was done, she came out again and asked how I was doing.

It was a fairly short period before the ambulance pulled up in front of the house. A person came to the front door and knocked, and Connie had let him in. He was there to assess the situation and quickly returned to the rig to get a gurney. Two men returned with the gurney, and they immediately put me on the gurney and took me out to the ambulance. Connie had also walked out with us. Addressing the ambulance driver, she said, "To Strong Memorial, please."

Strong was located in Rochester and was an excellent hospital for this type of thing. By this time, the pain had become very intense, and I wondered if I was having a heart attack. They closed the doors, and we were off to Rochester.

When we arrived at the hospital, I was taken into the emergency room. When the doctor came in, he ordered a blood pressure and some other quick tests be taken. They also gave me a shot for pain. After taking the blood pressure, they took me to the x-ray department to have films done. After they were done there, I was admitted to the hospital and taken to my floor.

Connie came into my room shortly after I was taken back. We had just begun talking when Dr. W, who was my heart doctor, walked in. Our conversation was cut short so Connie could talk with the doctor. Evidently, he had seen a growth on my lung that he was worried about. He decided to keep me in the hospital for a day or two to determine what it actually was and what should be done about it.

With the medication which they gave me, the pain had subsided. As a result, my neck and back began to hurt more because of the bed I had to lie on. It was very hard, which created big problems for my back.

People have no idea what a very hard bed can do to a bad back. You can feel anything that puts undo pressure to the back. My back was so sensitive that the pain just shot to my brain. Many times, people seemed to think that it was all in my head, but if they had to go through the same experience, they would quickly understand how bad it really was.

The day went by slowly, and Connie had gotten a phone hooked up and a TV for me to watch. I told her that she didn't have to stay any longer and could go home. I assured her I would be all right. Every time I had to go to the hospital and stay, I would say the same thing like a record. Connie was use to it and always thought I was trying to get rid of her, which was not the case at all. Connie was the type of person who would stay all night if she felt it was needed. She was a very caring person, and that's why I married her. She was just great through our marriage and took care of me all the time. Through our life together, I had been in the hospital many times and was aware of most of the procedures that happen during the course of the day.

The doctor came back into see me in the late afternoon. Connie had been gone for a while but had just returned to the room. He told the two of us that I had a pulmonary embolism that would have to be treated with blood thinners. I would be released the following day and would need to continue on the blood thinners until for a full week.

I woke up early the next morning and had my breakfast. Connie came about nine thirty, and I was dressed and ready to leave. I got checked out and wheeled to the car. I got in the car, and Connie drove home.

After my stay in the hospital, I got back into the therapy sessions twice a week. During the latter part of April and throughout May, I had several doctors' appointments. The discomfort in my neck remained painful, and when I saw Dr. B, I told him. However, he wanted me to continue without changing the strength of my pain patch yet. He wanted me to hold out as long as I could.

I knew I was taking enough of these very strong drugs, but I didn't know what to think anymore. I wish I knew when I would find a doctor to help me. Things were really driving me crazy. I didn't know what was going to happen with my life and wondered if I'd every work again. I prayed to God that he would give me an answer soon.

Fortunately, with all of my doctors in Batavia, we didn't have to worry about driving in the heavy Rochester traffic. The weather had been good throughout the past four or five months, which had been good for Connie. It didn't take a lot of time to get to appointments; the problem was that I had so many.

Along with all of these doctors' appointments, I also had to go to unemployment meetings so I could collect a check each month. This was a really demoralizing thing to do. The people whom you deal with make you feel like the money is coming out of their pockets. I really hated going to those meetings.

Our lives were quite busy, and I had hoped that no further problems would occur. I had been through enough and wanted no other medical problems in our family. I continued to hope that I would soon find out what the problem was with my damn neck. I was getting a very bad vibe that it may not happen. I remember thinking that I could not continue like this anymore. I was depressed and really wondered if I would ever be able to lead a little life again. I knew that Connie also felt really bad about everything, but there wasn't much we could do. My only hope was to find a good doctor who may be able to relieve my neck pain.

I was not able to make the appointment Connie had set up with the new psychiatrist because of my hospitalization. A new appointment was made, and I was looking forward to seeing the new doctor, as we had a lot to talk about. I felt a great relief knowing that I was going to get to unload all of my internal problems. I would meet with Dr. Le in two days.

Those couple of days went by quickly, and I was really looking forward to seeing Dr. Le. I had heard so many good things about him and was excited to sit down with him. Connie and I drove to Batavia and went into his office. Connie had to fill out some insurance information. After that was done, I was taken into his office. We shook hands, and I looked and was amazed to see that he had a big leather couch. I asked if I could lie down, and he said yes.

He began by asking me what had happened. I told him, and he asked me how I felt about the whole thing. I began to cry. He told me to get it off my chest. He said to me, "Things have been tough, haven't they?" I told him that they'd been very tough. He asked me how I felt mentally, and I told him very bad. We talked for about forty-five minutes. As we were wrapping up our session, he told me he was going to give me some pills that would help me get through the rough times. He gave me a prescription for lorazepam to calm me down when I became all excited. I thanked him, and he said he wanted to see me the following week. When I came out of the office, I thanked the receptionist for getting me in as a patient.

Connie and I left and got in the car for home. She asked me what I thought, and I told her he was great. When we got home, I took my normal place on the couch. My neck was hurting quite a bit, so I took a hydrocodone to take out some of the pain. I really hated taking the hydrocodone on top of the fentanyl patch, but I really needed it at times and didn't take that many. I lay down for a while and then got up and walked around. I went outside for a couple of minutes and then came back in and lay down. My problem was I could only stand up or lie down, so that's why I napped quite a bit.

The rest of the week was busy with physical therapy and getting blood work done. I then had to see my new psychiatrist. This was the normal schedule of each week. I was hopeful that Connie and I could get to the bottom of all of this, as I'd had so many tests that I don't even know why many of them were performed.

The following week, I had to see my pain specialist, along with Dr. L (my psychologist), and then Dr. Le (my psychiatrist). I was looking forward to seeing Dr. Le, as I felt myself becoming very depressedwith this pain I am dealing with. It had been so long, and I didn't know what to do. Maybe it would be better if I weren't alive any longer.

CHAPTER 9

On May 15, of 2001 I found myself outside enjoying the fairly nice weather. I was walking around looking at the house and assessing what had to be done for spring cleanup. Strolling down the street toward me was John, a good friend who was a patrolman for the local police department. He knew that I had fallen the year before and asked how I was.

I told him that my neck was really giving me a problem with a lot of pain, but my back didn't hurt all the time any longer. He told me about his mother who had been crippled for the past five years and who had been seeing a neurosurgeon in Rochester. The family were amazed at how the doctor had helped his mother with surgery.

John did tell me of one problem, though. He warned me that the doctor's office rescheduled appointments a lot. He gave me the doctor's name, and I thanked him very much. After he left, I went in and told Connie about our conversation. We both agreed that we would check into his background and then maybe call for an appointment.

I was very enthused that maybe we had found the doctor who would change my life around. I hoped that maybe he was the one who would find the problems I was having with my neck. I didn't understand why my back didn't hurt as much as it had in the beginning. At that point in time, I only felt it when I traveled in the car for long periods of time—then it was quite painful.

I was still going to physical therapy every other day and spending an hour there. I didn't know what it was doing for me, but I decided that I would continue to go. I was also continuing to see Dr. L and Dr. Le. I looked forward to my upcoming appointments with Dr. Le.

I didn't do much after physical therapy, as I was tired. Each day after therapy, I would lie down and fall asleep for an hour or two. On this particular day, nothing had changed. Connie had supper ready at five o'clock, and when we were done eating, I went to lie back down. I watched TV until eleven and then got ready for bed. While watching TV, I fell asleep and slept through the night.

The next morning, I woke up at eight o'clock and decided to take a ride to Ace Hardware to see my friends. My neck was not too bad that morning, but that had always been the way it was, and the pain always got worse as the day went on. I stayed at Ace for about an hour and then headed home.

I decided to lie down until we had to get ready for my appointment in Batavia. When we arrived at my appointment, my friend was waiting for me at the door. He opened the door for us, and Connie and I went in and sat down. We talked for an hour about things that had happened during the week. With Dr. L was always there for me when I needed someone to talk to quickly. He always made time for me, and I really respected him for that. He was a very nice guy.

After the appointment, Connie and I left and stopped at the restaurant to get something to eat. Connie was very surprised that I wanted to stop, but I felt she deserved it. She had been cooking meals for two weeks, and we didn't go out much at all. We only went out when I felt okay. We went in and had a good early dinner. I was up several times with my back, but still, Connie enjoyed the time out.

When we got home, I lay down and was quite tired. It was my intention to just lie down for an hour or so, but I ended up lying down for about four hours. I then had a problem getting to sleep at my normal time. I got ready for bed at midnight and didn't fall asleep until about one thirty. I was up at eight o'clock in the morning, and I just lay around until Connie got up at nine. Our appointment was at one thirty in Batavia. The morning went by slowly and we were ready to go by noon. Connie wanted to leave by one o'clock, and we did. We walked into the office twenty minutes later. Connie sat, and I paced. The doctor came through the door and asked me in.

When I went in, I took my position on the couch, and we began where we left off the previous week. I became very sentimental again as we talked about what had been happening. I told him that I'd been very depressed and thought about suicide a couple of times after Connie lost her job. Dr. Le was very compassionate toward what had been happening to us. He told me that he was going to work with me on building my self-esteem up again. He told me that it was going to take time, but he assured me that things would get better. He couldn't tell me how much better, but he stressed that I needed to have a positive attitude. I felt very good being with him. After the session, Connie and I drove home.

When we got home, we started to talk about the neurosurgeon my friend had told me about. I was ready to discover what the problem with my neck was. Connie agreed to call his office to get an appointment to see him. I remembered what John had told me about the office being so busy and often having to reschedule. I figured that if he was that busy, then he must have been good. Connie and I talked about the new specialist and both agreed that it was time to take care of this big problem that I was having. I'd had this pain long enough and needed to get it taken care of soon. I hoped and prayed that when the new doctor found the problem, if he could, that I would once again feel better. I hoped that someday I could return to work, but I didn't really know if that would be possible.

Connie didn't waste any time calling Dr. Z, the neurosurgeon in Rochester, for an appointment. She was given May 24, 2001, as the first available appointment date. I didn't think that was bad, as it was only a couple of weeks away, and I had already waited so long. Hopefully, my appointment didn't get rescheduled, and I would be able to see him as planned.

A couple of days later, I received a call from Dr. Z's office saying the appointment had to be rescheduled because he would be in surgery all day on the twenty-fourth. I then saw what John meant when he told me about the rescheduling. A new appointment was scheduled for June 12, 2001. At that point, things really got rough for me mentally, and I wondered if I'd ever be able to see him.

While waiting for my newly scheduled appointment with Dr. Z, I had to continue seeing all of my other doctors and going to the therapy sessions. Everything was becoming very boring, because I didn't feel that anything was helping my neck, or anything else for that matter. On top of all of that, I had to go to the unemployment bureau in Batavia to sign up for unemployment benefits. At times, I became confused as to what I should be doing. I knew the pain in my neck was getting a little stronger, so I was thankful to have the hydrocodone to help out.

CHAPTER 10

It was the day before Jenny graduated from college, which was a big event in our family. I hoped I would be able to attend the ceremony, but I knew it would depend on how I felt. I was so proud of my little girl, who was now all grown up. My life revolved around her; she was, and still is, the best daughter a father could ever have. She had never been a problem growing up, and she was about to become a nurse just like her mother.

In the beginning, Connie tried to talk Jenny out of becoming a nurse. Jenny was insistent, though, and I am so glad she was. I knew she would be a great nurse. She had studied very hard and deserved everything that was ahead of her. We were so proud of her.

When I got up the day of the graduation, I knew it was one of the two days a week I was free from all of my appointments. I felt pretty good and hoped I would be able to go to Jenny's graduation in Batavia that afternoon. My mom and sister would be attending, and I was excited to be able to have pictures of us all together.

After lying down during the morning for a while, I had some breakfast. I then walked around for a while to try and build myself up a little for the afternoon. We had to begin getting ready about one thirty, as the graduation began at four thirty. We got ready and left the house at three o'clock, so we would be able to find some good seats. That didn't matter to me, but my family had to sit down,

I started to experience more pain in my neck, so I took a hydrocodone, hoping to take care of the problem. We arrived at the college and parked the car. When we got to the entrance, my mom and sister Rozella were there waiting for us. We then went in and found our seats. We found a nice spot, so we were able to see everything. Of course, I was in the aisle standing up with my camcorder. The service took about an hour and a half, and seeing our daughter walk across the stage brought tears to my eyes. Our baby was all grown up and receiving her diploma to be a nurse. We were so proud of her.

Our house was set up by some friends for Jenny's graduation party. So when we arrived home, everything was ready for guests to arrive. My neck was still doing okay, and I hoped that I could get through the party and then go in to lie down later. Eventually, we had more than a hundred guests, and I believed that Jenny was very happy. The party lasted about three hours. When everyone was gone, Jenny decided to leave and go to a couple of other parties for her friends.

I helped clean up a little and then went in to lie down on the couch. My neck began to hurt more. I felt fortunate to have made it through everything, and I knew Jenny was very happy that I could. I was all washed up for the rest of the night. I got a little something to eat at about eight o'clock that evening, and then I was out like a light for the rest of the night.

I woke up Sunday morning and was still a little tired. I should have stayed in bed but decided to get up for the day instead. It was about nine o'clock, and I got some breakfast before going outside for a small walk. When I returned, I decided to lie on the couch but hoped I would not fall asleep. I wanted to be able to sleep that night, as the following day would be busy. I had physical therapy, blood work that had to be done, and a pain specialist appointment. I was going to talk with Dr. B about my pain problems with my neck. I had a feeling that if I began to make a big thing of my neck. I decided to wait till after I had seen the neurosurgeon—whenever I could get to see him. I hoped that I'd made the correct decision so I didn't end up in total pain.

Connie and I lay around during the day. We had an early dinner and watched TV for the rest of the night. I decided to go to bed at about ten o'clock, as I was a little tired from Saturday. I got dressed and went to lie down on the couch. Soon I had fallen to sleep, but Connie probably stayed up until one or two. in the morning.

I was up early in the morning at around six o'clock. I went outside to take a short walk. The weather wasn't too bad, so I must have walked for about an hour. Connie had gotten up at about ten o'clock, and I had a two o'clock appointment with my doctor. From there, I had to go to the hospital to have some blood work done. Connie had gotten something to eat and then got into the shower. When she was done, I got in. It was about one fifteen when we left for Batavia.

I walked into the doctor's reception area and signed in. Connie then sat down, and I paced as usual. About five minutes later, the girl came and took Connie and me into the waiting room. Shortly after that, the doctor walked in and asked how I was doing. I told him that I was doing fine. I told him about the appointment with the neurosurgeon in Rochester. He was glad that I'd found another doctor and wished me luck. After the meeting with the doctor, Connie and I drove to the hospital so I could have my blood work done. After this was done, we drove home and ordered a pizza for dinner so Connie wouldn't have to cook.

My week ahead was going to be quite busy with therapy sessions and then seeing Dr. L near the end of the week. The time went by quickly, and before I knew, it I was ready for my physical therapy visit on Monday morning. At my appointment, I had to lie face down on a long table while the therapist massaged my neck. As I lay there, he began to massage my neck. He wasn't even pushing hard when, all of a sudden, I let out a very loud scream of pain. Evidently, he had hit the bad nerve in my neck, and the tears began rolling down my cheeks. I couldn't believe how bad the pain felt. It was an excruciating pain that I'd never felt before. The therapist immediately said that he didn't push hard, and I told him that I knew he hadn't. I realized that I couldn't go on any longer and decided to leave. The therapist asked if I was okay, and I told him yes and drove home. When I got home, Connie wondered what the problem. I told her and then went to lie down on the couch.

After I was settled, Connie told me that Dr. Z's office called to reschedule my appointment again. It was now rescheduled from June 12 to June 16, which was a Saturday. After listening to Connie, I decided to take a hydrocodone for pain. After lying back down, I fell asleep. When I woke up, I decided to cancel the rest of the therapy sessions for the week, along with my appointment with Dr. L. Connie had waited until morning to make the calls to cancel my appointments. My neck was still hurting to some extent. This was by far the worse pain I'd felt in my neck since I'd fallen in October 2000.

I knew that I needed to get to see Dr. Z as soon as I could. I had to see him, as I was really worried that something may happen to cripple me. All it would take was having something hit wrong. The days went very slowly, and my neck did not fully heal. Each day I would touch the area the therapist had been rubbing with his fingers and felt a slight feeling of pain. Each day I lay around the house instead of going out.

Finally, it was the Saturday of my appointment with Dr. Z. We got up and got ready for the trip to Rochester. We had to leave at noon to be there on time.

We got into the car and took off for Rochester. We knew right where his office was located. As we pulled into the parking lot, I noticed that there were several cars there. I wondered if the cars all belonged to patients of Dr. Z or if there were other doctors in the same office. As we walked through the door with his name on it, we entered a very large room. It was almost the size of a half court in basketball. It was very large with probably thirty people in there. Some wore neck braces, while others had canes. After looking around the waiting room, I understood why they rescheduled so much. This doctor had to be really good.

Connie and I went to the window, and I signed in. In turn, I was handed a bunch of papers to fill out. Connie took them and sat down in a chair. I walked up and down the aisle. After about twenty minutes, Connie had finished with the papers. I walked them up to the window and also handed the receptionist my insurance cards. After making copies of the cards, she returned them to me. We remained in the room for another ten minutes before our name was called to follow a young lady to a room.

We walked with her to the waiting room, and Connie sat down. About five minutes later, this huge man at about six four and 280 pounds walked through the door and introduced himself. We, in turn, did the same. He began by asking why we were there to see him. I explained what had happened to me over the past eight months and told the story of how I'd just been to therapy where a very soft spot in my neck had been touched. The doctor was amazed that I had been through all of my history over the past eight months with no pain relief.

Dr. Z suggested that I have an MRI and a few other tests so he could reevaluate the results and make a determination of what to do. He asked about my back, and I told him that it hurt every once in a while but my neck was by far the most painful. We bid farewell, and Connie and I left to make another appointment and get prescriptions for the tests the doctor had recommended.

We met with Dr. Z's scheduler, and she gave us all the prescriptions and the date for the next appointment. Our next date to see him was July 7, 2001, at eight thirty in the morning. The appointment time was really early, but it was the quickest he could see me.

I continued with physical therapy, my pain specialist, and the psychologist for the next couple of weeks. I made sure at therapy that there was no massaging near the spot the therapist had touched before. I had to see the pain specialist in a couple of days, along with Dr. L. On Thursday, I had to go to Rochester for my MRI and a set of x-rays. My appointments with therapy were very light, as I wasn't going to take any chances before I saw Dr. Z again in a few days. I was hoping that at this next appointment he could do something for me. Connie and I picked up the results of the MRI and the x-rays to take with us on Saturday. We had to get up at four thirty in the morning, so Connie would have enough time to get ready.

We needed to leave at seven thirty to be there at eight thirty. Before we knew it, we were on the road to Rochester.

We arrived at eight fifteen and walked into the office. There weren't many people there, and we were in the waiting room for about five minutes after signing in. Then, through the door, Dr. Z walked in. Connie handed him the tests results, and he began to look at the info right away. He then looked at me and said that I needed to have surgery performed on my neck.

He explained that he needed to perform a fusion in my neck and install a steel plate with four screws. I began to cry, and I was sure he wondered why. But he looked at me and fully understood why I was crying. He said to me, "I know that you have been through a lot of pain for a long time, and now we will take care of it for you."

I asked myself why no one else could see what he saw. I wanted to know why I had to suffer for so long. I could not believe that things would finally be taken care of. Another appointment needed to be scheduled before we could proceed.

I had to see my heart specialist to have a stress test and blood work done. I also had to continue with my therapy appointments, see my pain specialist, and deal with unemployment and whatever else before I went under the knife. My next appointment with Dr. Z was on July 31, 2001. At that time, we would confirm all of the things I needed done. With all of the meetings I had with doctors, unemployment, and everything else, I prayed that I could have the surgery done soon.

On July 24, I woke up with chest pains again and was very worried about the problem. I had seen my heart specialist, and all was well. He felt I was just worried about all that was to happen soon. Finally, our day to see Dr. Z had arrived. We had to be at his office at nine thirty, and we were in the car at eight thirty. We arrived at his office and went into the waiting room right away. The doctor walked in and wanted to make sure all was taken care of, and I was set to have surgery. I had all the blood work done, as well as stress tests and other things. I was ready.

Dr. Z finally told us he would operate on August 27. We had to call for pre-op testing, and we'd receive the time of surgery. I had to quit smoking for one month prior to the surgery. What a shock this was, but I stopped right away. We were all done and left, and I was so happy.

I couldn't help but wonder why it was that no one believed me in the beginning. I could have committed suicide, and then what would have happened? Connie would have sued someone. In any event, the surgery was going to be done now. When we got home, I called my mom and my sister Rozella to tell them it was almost set. I was so happy, but I had to make sure that nothing would happen in the meantime to change everything.

CHAPTER 11

The time went by very slowly. I still had to do everything, including physical therapy and other doctors' appointments, before that special day came. Some nights I could not sleep because I couldn't stop thinking everything that was going on, but I knew it was finally going to be taken care of.

Finally, the day of pretesting had come, and we had to be there at twelve thirty that afternoon. When Connie and I arrived, we talked about all that was to happen. We would need to wait until the next day to find out what time the surgery would be. I was becoming very excited that this would be all over.

The weekend arrived, and I decided to take it easy and do nothing. Soon, it would be over. It was finally Sunday, and I realized that my surgery was scheduled on our anniversary August 27, which was tomorrow.. So many things had been going on that Connie and I had both forgot. I decided that the operation would be a great present. I had to be at the hospital at six o'clock in the morning, and my surgery was scheduled for nine o'clock. I went to bed early, as I hoped Connie would. I woke up once at about three o'clock to go to the bathroom and noticed a light in Connie's room. I didn't bother her and went back to sleep. I don't think she slept at all worrying about me.

I finally woke up at five thirty and went into Connie's room to wake her up. I was very nervous and hoped all of my misery would be over soon. We both got ready and left. We arrived a little early at the hospital, and I was really worried about the surgery, which was scheduled to begin just over an hour later. I had hoped to God I felt better when the surgery was done. I was taken to my room and prepped for the IV and whatever else had to happen.

Finally, it was time. I kissed Connie and told her I loved her. They wheeled me into the operating room where they gave me a shot through my IV, and I was out. My mom and my sister Rozella had come to the hospital after I was taken back for surgery.

The surgery took about four hours. When the doctors were done, I was wheeled into the recovery room. There they put my neck collar on, which I would have to wear for a couple of weeks to make sure I didn't hurt my neck. It was kind of heavy but really protected my neck fully. About an hour later, I was taken to my room. I was still very groggy but was able to talk to Connie. Not long after that, I was also able to see my mom and sister.

My neck hurt quite a bit, but I felt confident that it would be much better than before the surgery. I remember that there was one thing I did notice, and that was my back. It hurt an awful lot, but I had soon forgotten about it. A few hours later, Dr. Z walked in to check on me. He wanted to make sure I was all right. Dr. Z had spent a few minutes talking with Connie. He told her that he fused the C-5 C-6-C-7 vertebrae with a steel plate and screws and said he would check back a few hours later to see how I was doing.

He gave Connie specific instructions that I had to be very careful and wasn't to take off my neck brace for the first week. Connie had told him that I would keep the neck brace on and wouldn't begin to wash my neck until after the first week. We had a follow-up appointment at his office a week later. Connie said good-bye to Dr. Z as he walked out the door.

Soon, a nurse came in to get me up and moving around. I really didn't feel like it, but they wanted me to get up on my feet. When I slid off of the bed, my back really hurt, and I wondered what the hell was going on. It seemed that now I had more pain to deal with, and here I'd been thinking

I would be pain free. I had forgotten about the pain in my back, and it was really painful.

I finally got on my feet and began walking. The pain in my back had taken over any pain I first felt in my neck. I kept walking, and the nurse said that I was going to have to get up and walk around several times that day, as I would be going home the following day. I really wanted to go home, but I wondered what was going to happen with my back.

Dr. Z and I hadn't even talked about that, as I hadn't realized that I had any pain in my back. My neck pain was so bad I hadn't even thought to talk to Dr. Z about my back. The pain was all in my neck.

After about ten minutes of walking, I got back in bed and told Connie how bad my back was. I knew that there wasn't anything that could be done at the moment and hoped maybe it really wouldn't get that bad after all. Standing on my feet was creating a huge problem. I couldn't stand up for too long, as my spine was really hurting very badly. I realized I would have to be careful standing.

As I laid my head down on the pillow, I felt the pain in my neck. My back felt much better lying down. I soon fell asleep and was able to rest for about an hour. I woke up wondering at first where I was, but then I felt my neck and remembered. Connie was dozing in the chair nearby, and I know that she was quite tired. As soon as I moved, Connie opened her eyes and woke up. I told her I was sorry for waking her up. When she woke up, she said to me, "Happy Anniversary." I just laughed. What a day for surgery. I couldn't even take her out to dinner to celebrate this special occasion.

Soon, the nurse came around again, and I was able to take my next walk. Unfortunately, my neck hurt, but my back actually hurt much worse. At one point, I asked God why it was that I had to suffer so much through all of this. Going into the operation, I thought I would feel a lot better, but I realized how wrong I'd been. I couldn't help but wonder what I had done to deserve all of this. I was sure Connie was letting this go through her mind and asking the same question to God.

The night went fairly slowly. It was about nine o'clock pm when I asked Connie to leave. She didn't want to, but I talked her into it. I didn't like her driving in the dark, as her eyes were not the best, but she wouldn't admit it. She finally decided to go and gave me a kiss. I was so happy that she had stayed with me all day, but I was also really looking forward to going home the next day. I decided that I wouldn't worry about my back until I got home. Connie waved good-bye and walked out the door. After she left, I quickly fell asleep. I woke up again about midnight to go to the bathroom and then when back to bed.

I woke up several times during the night because of the pain I was having in my neck. However, the pain was not as bad as it had been leading up to this surgery. The next thing I remembered from that night was being woken up at four o'clock in the morning by the nurses so they could give me some pills. I then woke up at seven o'clock due to the shift change. I was looking forward to going home later in the day.

The pain I was experiencing in my back was always in the back of my mind. I decided that I would let God take care of everything. He wouldn't let me suffer too much. The phone rang at about nine o'clock, and it was Connie. She asked how I was and told me she would be over around eleven. I thanked her, blew her a kiss, and hung up.

Shortly after hanging up the phone, Dr. Z walked into the room and asked how I was doing. I told him my neck felt much better but explained that my back was now really bothering me. He told me that was a separate issue we had to take care of. He told me to have Connie call for an appointment in a week so he could check everything. I told him I would and then thanked him.

Just after I talked with Dr. Z, a nurse came in and took me for a walk to make sure all was okay. I had finished my breakfast just before Connie called and I had to go to the bathroom, so I had to make my walk fairly short. As I was walking, the pain going through my back was quite bad. I wondered how long it would last. I just couldn't get the pain in my backoff of my mind. After our walk, I immediately went into the bathroom. I had just made it and really felt relieved. I then went to my bed and pushed the button for the nurses' station. They replied to my signal, and I asked if I could take a shower. I had completely forgotten that I'd had neck surgery and wasn't supposed to shower for at least ten days. I was not about to try to get into a bathtub, and the nurses wouldn't let me anyway. Instead, I freshened up as well as I could, got dressed, and then waited for Connie to come. It was about eleven o'clock when she walked through the door. Now that I was ready to leave, I found that my neck brace was really hard to get used to.

The nurse came in with all of the papers for release. While Connie took care of the paperwork, a wheelchair was ordered to take me to the car. Connie took care of signing me out and went after the car. She met me in the exit area for patient pickup, and the nurse helped me into the car. I thanked her, and we left. I asked Connie if she was given the directions about what I should and shouldn't do, and she said that she had. Connie took off on the way to Le Roy.

We got home in about forty-five minutes, and I was happy to be there. However, when I got out of the car, my back was killing me. The pain was so bad getting out of car that a tear actually slid down my cheek. I knew that I was going to have some problems, but I would just have to handle it and then talk to Dr. Z at my appointment the following week.

I got into the house with Connie's help and immediately sat down on the couch. I was going to be really careful trying to lie down. I waited for Connie to bring in everything from the car and then asked her to help me lie down. The neck brace was very cumbersome, but I managed to lie down okay. Connie called Dr. Z's office and got an appointment for me on September 11, 2001, at one o'clock.

The next few days went fairly well. I had to be very careful of my neck, and I was not going to screw up the good job the doctor had done. On about the forth day, I really began to get very used to the neck brace and was able to do a few things around the house. I was also able to get up, walk around, and lie down again. My orders were very strict. I did have a chance to have a bath but had to be very careful. This was the first time I'd had a bath in about five years. I really felt clean when I was done, and Connie had to help me with everything. The only thing I did was sit there on a waterproof pillow. With my back the way it was, I needed it to sit, and even then, I couldn't stay in there too long.

My sister Rozella and mom called me not long after I'd gotten out of the tub. It was great hearing from the both of them. My sister Rozella had been taking care of our mom ever since I'd been hurt. I used to go to the house to take care of the outside. Now Rozella had to take care of everything, as if she didn't have enough to do with her kids and her house. In any event, I realized what a great family we had. I loved them all so much.

My appointment was with Dr. Z in a couple of days, and Mom and Rozella were coming to see me that day. I couldn't wait. I had a BM before they came, and it was very pain full in my back.

They stopped in about one o'clock and sat down, while I lay on the couch. Mom was doing just fine, and Rozella also was good. My family was so close, and we love each other so very much. They left about an hour later.

My appointment with Dr. Z was in two days, with my back problems, I really wanted to talk with him. We had to go into Rochester the next day to get films done of my neck so we could bring them to the appointment. Time had passed fairly quickly and before I knew it, the day of my appointment had arrived.

CHAPTER 12

At eight o'clock on the morning of September 11, 2001, I was preparing for my appointment with Dr. Z. I made sure Connie was up, as we had to be at the doctors at one o'clock that afternoon. I was walking around with my brace still on and hoped that I would be able to take the brace off at my appointment.

My neck felt just great, but my back was a different story. I continued to believe that it would get better over time.

As I was walking to the garage, I heard a horn honk and saw it was my good friend Frank D. He pulled up close to me and then turned the car off and got out. He wanted to know how I was doing. I was glad to see him, as I hadn't seen him in quite some time. We went into the house and chatted for about an hour and then walked out the front door. Connie had just come out from the bedroom and said good-bye to Frank.

As Frank and I were on the sidewalk out front, Connie hollered out the front door. She said that the World Trade Center had been hit by a plane. We were in total astonishment and immediately went into the house. Just as we got through the front door, another plane had crashed into the other building. It was like we were in a dream. We couldn't believe what we were watching—America was being attacked. But by whom, we didn't know. This was very serious, and I didn't know if I should cry or get mad. I got really mad and then thought about our appointment as to whether we should cancel. We decided not to. Frank left a short time after coming into the house.

I couldn't stop thinking about the Trade Centers and wondering about what was happening in America. I hadn't even thought of all the people who had been killed that day. But it was thousands of poor Americans are who were not to blame. It was hard to imagine what had created this massive kill by crazy people abducting airplanes. People cried all over the world that day. Connie and I went through the rest of that day in a daze over what had happened. America had been attacked by terrorists, and no one knew who they were or whom they represented. Pres. George W. Bush was at a school full of kids whom he was talking to when he received the news. The look on his face was total astonishment, and he quietly left at an opening in the program. God Bless all the people who lost their lives today.

After hearing the news of the attacks, I became very upset. I was crying about all of the pain I had, while many people had just lost their lives. I wondered what the hell was wrong with me. Didn't I have any sympathy for the human life? I was so upset with myself and made the decision to begin treating the situation the way it should be treated—with complete sympathy for everyone involved with this unheard of attack. The more I thought about it, the more I realized what an asshole I was. I could not believe my attitude about myself I was sure I would get over it, but in the meantime, I thought, *God, please forgive me.*

Connie and I still had to see my doctor that afternoon in Rochester. The appointment was at two thirty if he didn't reschedule it. We started to get ready at eleven thirty. When I got done washing up, as I still could not take a shower, Connie started to get ready while I watched the news regarding this awful attack. When she got out of the shower, the phone rang, and it was my mom. She had been watching it on TV and was all upset. Evidently, Rozella had walked in the door while she was talking with me. Rozella got on the phone for a minute and was also very upset. Who wouldn't be? Mom was also calling to see how I was. I told her I didn't know after this major event. She asked about my appointment, and I told her we had to be there at two thirty. We talked for a while, and then she had to go. I told her I loved her, and she hung up.

I sat down and watched the TV until Connie told me we were ready to leave. I had quickly finished dressing and made sure my neck brace was okay, and then I got into the car. It took about forty minutes to get to Dr. Z's office. When I got out of the car, my back hurt an awful lot, and I had to walk around outside for about five minutes before I went inside to sign in. Once again, there were many patients there to see the doctor.

Connie sat down, and I paced around for about fifteen minutes before we were called in. Several people were staring at me with my neck brace on. There were a few people who also had neck braces on when we went into the waiting room. Connie had just sat down and I'd begun to walk around, when Dr. Z came through the door. He wanted to know how I was doing with my neck, and I told him good. He looked at the films and was very happy with the healing of my neck. After looking at the films, I told him how bad my back was.

He looked at me and kind of laughed and then said that he was not surprised. When I had told him about my neck hurting very badly and how I could feel my back at times, he knew that my neck was over shadowing my back pain. He had guessed that when he fixed my neck, my back would take over with all of the pain. This almost knocked me over. He had known all along what the outcome was going to be. Connie and I looked at each other and kind of laughed. Dr. Z mentioned he wanted me to continue with physical therapy and come back to see him in a month so he could reevaluate my back. I also had to have another MRI for my back and x-rays of my neck before going back. He also told me I could take my neck brace off. We thanked him and left.

Connie and I had to see Dr Z on September 15, 2001. I was still to take it easy, but I could now take showers. I thought that was great. I was still watching the TV regarding the September 11 massacre of America. I still could not believe my eyes. We found out that a family down the street from us lost a granddaughter who worked in the Twin Towers and went to Le Roy High School. That was when it began to really hit home.

As the days went by, my neck felt much better. The neurosurgeon had found the problem in my neck and had taken care of it. I began hoping that he would soon think about taking care of my back. He had already said that from looking at the films of my back, he was not ready to do any surgery yet. I began to fear what was going to be done to my back and when.

I was still going to my regular therapy along with seeing Dr. Z and Dr. B. Seeing Dr. Le always was a good get-together for me. He could really open me up with all of my problems. I sure had a full schedule to try and rebuild my body. The therapy would become difficult at times, but the people working with me really cared about me and tried their best to get me back on my feet with strength. I hoped our work there would help me in the end. Dr. B also helped me quite a bit. The patch would now have to fight the pain of my back. I was hopeful that it would continue to help me until Dr. Z was ready to do the surgery.

The next few days were quite busy. I would definitely have welcomed a good break. I was really going to take it easy. On September 13, 2001, I had nothing to do. I was able to just lie around. I enjoyed just watching TV. My back was okay as long as I was lying down.

Connie made a great pizza for dinner that night, and I really looked forward to that. After dinner, we watched TV, and I went to bed at about eleven o'clock. I only woke up once that night to go to the bathroom. I then slept till nine o'clock in the morning, which was a long time for me. My back really hurt when I got up, so I decided to lie down instead of going out.

I stayed around the house that day as well and did nothing. Connie had gotten up at about eleven o'clock that morning, and I was watching TV. She had decided to do the laundry, and I went into my bedroom to get all my clothes ready for the wash. After I got them ready, I was walking into the living room when a very sharp pain went down the front of my leg. The pain was very bad, and it was the first time I had that type of pain in a very long time.

In fact, the last time I'd experienced such pain was before my back surgery in 1986. Then I had the back surgery, and the pain was gone for what I thought was forever. How wrong I was. I realized at that moment that I was going to really have to take care. I immediately went to lie down on the couch and told Connie about the pain I had. I ended up lying on the couch until dinner. We didn't even know what we were going to have, but I knew we wouldn't starve. We had decided to buy our food out, and I would bring it home.

At about five thirty that evening, I got up and felt no pain like I'd experienced earlier. I told Connie that I would go and pick some food up for us to eat. Connie thought that sounded great, and I decided to go to Burger King, as we had not eaten anything from there for a long time. I picked up a couple of cheeseburgers and got some fries before heading back home. When I got home, we both sat down and ate. It was good for a while for me, and then the pain in my leg started up again. I was so depressed that I had to fight this pain again. I went through the same thing with my neck for a long time, and now I was going through it with my back.

I really had thoughts of possibly going back to work again. I was only fifty-five at the time and could have worked another ten to fifteen years if I were healthy. Of course, I wasn't healthy. I was hoping that when I had my back surgery, I would once again feel much better. I knew I needed to talk to Dr. Z to see what the story was.

It seemed that we could not get a break at all. Things seemed to have just gotten worse since I'd fallen. Nothing really good had happened to us since my fall. We had nothing at all to be happy about. I kept wondering what I'd done to create such a negative life for both Connie and me.

CHAPTER 13

After deciding to get ready for bed early one night, I went to take my spot on the couch and watch TV until I fell asleep. I gave Connie a kiss instead and fell asleep. I watched TV until about midnight, but I must have dozed off. I must have been fairly tired, as I don't remember getting up in the middle of the night at all. I woke up at seven in the morning and decided to hang around the house for a while before going to get the papers. I had started to play the lottery a few weeks earlier and really looked forward to checking the numbers to see if I'd won.

Well, I checked the numbers a little later after getting the papers. I wasn't a winner, and I wasn't even close. That seemed to be the norm twice a week when I bought the tickets. In the past, I had won $500 and $1,750, but that was long ago. My luck has not been good at all for a long time.

After my loss again, I walked outside a little to loosen up my back. It hurt quite a bit, but I had taken a hydrocodone a while ago, so it wasn't as bad as it could have been. I really hated having to live on the pain pills, but there was nothing I could do about it. The fentanyl I still took was also strong, but I needed all of this medication to survive. I started out with 25 micrograms and it I was beginning to feel like I wasn't worth anything anymore, as I could not do anything. I had been through my neck problem not really knowing about my back. I felt stupid not to even consider this, but things could have been worse. I could have been dead after I'd fallen down the stairs at work.

I went into the house around nine fifteen that morning, and just as I took my coat off, the phone rang. I hurried to pick it up, as I didn't want Connie to hear it and wake up. It was my niece Carol on the phone, and I asked how she was. She told me that the ambulance had taken my sister Rozella into the hospital at seven o'clock that morning. Carol, who was Rozella's twin daughter, called to let me know. I told her I would call my sisters, but she had already called them both. I thanked her for calling me and then became very excited, so I took a lorazepam to help me calm down. What else could happen to Connie and me? Rozella had been to see me at the hospital many times and always looked after me. I loved her so much. I waited for Connie to wake up, and then we would decide what to do.

When she got up, we sat down and talked about the whole situation with Rozella and the family. We had been down for so long, and this was another major blow to us. Our family was so tight, and Connie and I had to go to Rochester to see her if we could. We decided to go. My back would really take a large hit riding in a car for that long, but I had to do it to go see my sister.

We both got ready and left at about one thirty for Rochester. On the way, I changed positions in the car several times due to my back. It took us about forty-five minutes to get there. When I got out of the car, I was all crippled up and had to walk around for a while to loosen up as best I could. We walked into the lobby, and the family was there talking and walking around. I saw my niece Carol and asked how her mother was. She told us that she was confused, but we would be able to see her for a short time.

Connie and I went upstairs in the elevator with Carol. She was very upset but was handling the situation as well as she could. On our way up to Rozella's room, Carol told us what had happened. Apparently, she had gotten up very early in the morning. Her husband, Ed, asked what was wrong, but he wasn't awake enough to realize there was a problem. It wasn't until six o'clock that morning when Rozella was up again that he realized something was seriously wrong. It turned out that she'd had a stroke sometime during the night.

I was really nervous about seeing her in a different manor than she normally was. When we walked in, she saw me, and I sat on the bed with her. I had a beard at the time, and she kept rubbing my beard laughing. We stayed for only about fifteen minutes before we had to leave. I kissed her several times, and then we went back downstairs. I didn't know it at the time, but that would be the last time I saw her alive. We spoke to other family members in the waiting room for twenty minutes or so and then left for home. A few days later, Rozella passed away.

I took her death very hard. This was the sister who took care of me so much in my life. She was sixteen years older than me—almost old enough to be my mother. Many times earlier in life, she would wheel me around in my baby carriage. She took me everywhere with her, and many people thought I was her baby. She filled my life with joy and did the same for everyone else she came in contact with.

After Rozella's death, my other sisters flew in from Connecticut and Colorado with their families. We were all at the funeral. I could not spend much time at the service because of my back, but I was there much longer than I thought I would be. I kissed her for the last time, and the tears came running down my cheeks as I told her how much I loved her. Rozella died on September 22, 2001.

Some of the family stayed a couple of days after the funeral. I really felt bad because the funeral was on my sister Sharon's birthday. What a memory she will have about the day of the funeral. My birthday was on September 30. The month of September would be remembered for many years to come due to September 11, 2001, and to our family it would be remembered also.

I had wondered how many more bad things would happen to Connie and me. I still think it would have been so easy if I had never gotten up from that fall I had. Sure, it would have been tough on Connie, Jenny, and my family for a while, but they wouldn't have had to put up with me.

We had been through so much. I was never so much concerned with myself, but my wife and daughter have had to go through so many things with me. Connie's life had been ruined along with mine. She hadn't been able to do anything outside of the house other than get groceries. Her life had completely stopped for me, as she was by my side all of the time. I often wondered how much longer I would have to go through all of this pain crap and hoped it would be over soon.

CHAPTER 14

October 1, 2001, finally arrived. One year had passed since my fall, and the problem still hadn't been fully taken care of. I really began to wonder if I would ever go back to work. We were getting by, but who knew for how long. That week I had an appointment with the lawyers representing me in my civil lawsuit. I knew it would last a long time, but I would worry about that later on in life.

I also had to see Dr. L that same week and have a CAT scan. I didn't have any physical therapy the whole month of October.

My appointments with my pain specialist were also very light that month, and Dr. Z was beginning to become more concerned about my back. He ordered more tests, and I hoped that the surgery would take place fairly soon. God knows I was ready, as no one should have to live through the pain that I'd lived with for the past year.

My life hadn't been worth a shit, and I had ruined Connie's life, along with the lives of the rest of my family. It seemed that anything that came up for us to do always turned out very bad. For example, when we were asked to friends' houses, I would end up leaving very quickly. It put us in a very bad situation.

I'm sure there were times when Connie wondered how bad my back really was. More than once, we had planned something because I was feeling fairly good. Connie would spend time getting ready, and then by the time we were ready to leave, I no longer felt good. I hated for this to happen, but I couldn't help it.

My pain often increased or decreased without warning. This had been going on for a long time, and it had finally resulted in us not doing anything any longer. This began to create problems with our marriage, but there was nothing I could do. The pain had taken over my life and my mind. Because I found myself wondering if my life would ever get better again, I began having deeper mental problems. I was having thoughts that things would not turn out good at all. I prayed to God that this would not be the case.

I had already scheduled all of my appointments for the month. Though it was a light month, I was still very tired with a lot of pain. The fentanyl patch had helped, but the remaining pain was still very bad. I didn't know what to do any longer. I had no other direction to go, and it was not worth going through all of this any longer.

Connie and I hadn't had sex for more than a year at this point. I wouldn't even go into her room to snuggle like we use to do. I was so afraid of straining my back and even my neck, although it felt a lot better. I couldn't take even a small chance, as I feared the outcome could be much worse. I realized that any more pain would give me serious thoughts about ending my life. I just couldn't take any more.

I wished that Connie really understood me more than she did. I was kind of surprised that she didn't, but there was nothing I could do to change how she felt or even thought.

I just hoped the pain would get better at some point in time. I realized that our marriage would never be what it was before I got hurt.

I had still been thinking about my sister being gone, but nothing I said or did was going to bring her back. I would pray, *God, please watch over my older sister, and I thank you, Rozella, for all the times you spent with me. I love you so much, and I miss you so much already.* I knew that life must go on, and I hoped I would be able to handle everything coming my way.

I owed it to the lady who had taken care of me every day since I'd been hurt. Connie didn't deserve this, but there was nothing I could do. Maybe, someday, I would be able to try and pay her back somehow.

I had tried to go over to see my brother-in-law Ed who had taken the death of my sister very hard. He felt that his life was basically over. He didn't realize how much he cared for her. She was everything to him, but he worked so hard to support his family that it was hard for him to distinguish the difference between working hard all of the time and spending quality time with Rozella.

I wasn't able to do anything since I'd been injured. It was suggested to me by a friend to go to the nursing home to visit people. I thought about this for a few minutes and didn't know if I wanted to do this. I figured I would think about it for a day or two.

My back pain was really getting to me. When I didn't feel good, I would sometimes take it out on Connie. I knew that she didn't deserve it, but there was nothing I could do.

At times, I had thought about trying to get involved with a group of people who were all dealing with severe back pain. But what would it really do for me? It wouldn't cut my pain at all. However, it might take my mind off of the pain I was living with. If I were to stand up and tell other individuals about the pain I had, they would understand. We would all be talking about something that everybody understood. After thinking it over, I decided that may not be a bad idea and resolved to look into it to see what I could find.

On November 30, 2001, I decided that I was going to go over to the nursing home. I was not worried about going into the building and just introducing myself. A lot of people become very scared trying to do something like this, but I was not. I knew that in some cases I would be talking to some people who didn't have anyone come to visit them. I figured that maybe I could really help some of these people out, and it may even make me feel better trying to help someone else. I decided to mention it to Connie and told her I that I would be going the next morning, which was Monday. It couldn't be a better day to start.

I watched TV for a while after dinner that night and thought I would go to bed a little early, as I was a little tired. When I went to bed, I decided to watch TV. I remember having to go to the bathroom, and when I got up, it was four o'clock in the morning, and I had slept fairly soundly. At times, I had big problems trying to get back to sleep, but on that particular morning, I was pretty tired so I went right back to sleep. My back was bothering me a little, but I was so tired I still went right back to sleep.

I woke up at about eight o'clock and thought about the nursing home. I decided that I would go about ten thirty or eleven. I thought it would be best to get into the shower before Connie got up. I thought that she was up quite late reading the night before, so she might not be up until eleven thirty or so. My back was bothering me quite a bit, but I began to think about the people at the home. I couldn't remember if we had relatives there or not, but I figured that I'd soon find out.

My back was really giving me some problems, but what else was new. The pain just hung on and wouldn't let go. I now fully understood in life what people go through living with pain every single day. It ruins everything in a person's life. I could see that my marriage was becoming affected by all of this. I didn't want to hurt anyone over things like this, but I couldn't help it. Every minute of every day was pain. I had these strong patches on my shoulder, I knew that they were helping me, but the left over pain was just awful. I prayed to God, asking him what I had done to offend him and make him so mad as to let something like this happen to me. I had always been nice to people and been very courteous, but it still happened.

When I got out of the shower, it was a little after nine o'clock, and I had to be careful while drying my back and also drying my legs and feet. I couldn't bend over well, and if I did, it really hurt. I finally got dried off and did all the usual things to get ready for the day. By the time I left the house, it was nearly ten, and I decided to leave a note for Connie just in case she forgot I was going to the nursing home.

I drove uptown for a few minutes to get gas. My back was pretty good in the car for about thirty minutes before it really got bad. The model car we drove was not good for anyone with a bad back. I swore that if we could ever afford it, we would get a bigger car that I could sit in and feel pretty good.

I arrived at the parking lot of the nursing home and pulled in. I got out of the car and walked through the front door where I was greeted by a receptionist. She asked what she could help me with, and I told her that I was there to visit. She asked me who, and I told her everyone. She really thought that was nice to come over to see the people there. I asked her if she knew of anyone there who didn't have any relatives or friends who came to see them. She gave me a couple of names, and that's where I stopped first.

I first met a man who had been there about three months while recovering from a heart attack. He had no one who came to see him. I introduced myself and began talking with him. His wife had died a few years earlier, and they had no kids. He lived in Batavia and was a janitor for one of the middle schools up until he'd gotten sick. I visited with him for about forty-five minutes, just talking about everything. He gave me the impression that he was a very likeable person but was very nervous talking to other people. I decided that I'd make sure to see him each time I came to visit. When I left the room, my back was really giving me a lot of pain. I couldn't sit, so I had been on my feet for nearly an hour, and the throbbing was becoming stronger.

I decided to see just one more person. I began walking the halls when I noticed Connie's aunt was sitting in a wheelchair down the hallway. I walked down there and began to talk with her. Her name was Onalee, and she was just a wonderful lady. I always liked her and her husband, Cliff. They always treated me very nicely. She had been in the nursing home for quite some time, but I wasn't really sure what her problem was. I would ask Connie when I got home. We chatted for about half an hour when I told her I had to leave but would see her again soon. I gave her a kiss and said good-bye to her.

I walked out of the building and drove the five minutes home. When I walked in the back door, I noticed that the coffee maker had not been started yet, which told me Connie wasn't up yet. Soon after I closed the back door, Connie came walking into the kitchen. She was still kind of sleeping, so we did little talking until she woke up fully. I decided to go into the living room and lie down for a while, as my back and neck were hurting quite a bit. I just put my head on the pillow, and before I knew it, I had fallen asleep. I must have been there for about an hour before I got up.

I felt a little refreshed and decided that I would create a new book about the drugs I was taking. This would be a book I would use to record times I took each drug so I didn't take anything twice. I sat down on my couch with a pillow under my butt, a ruler in my hand, and a new logbook on the table in front of me. With supplies ready, I began making a logbook. Over the past few months, I had forgotten what drugs I took and when, so I figured this was the best thing to do.

Fortunately, I wasn't taking a lot of drugs at that particular time, so I only had a few to keep track of. Even so, I didn't want to take the wrong pills at the wrong times. That scared me. Over the next few years, it did happen on a couple of occasions. Fortunately, it didn't create any big problems, but it frightened me nonetheless. I had always been afraid of taking very strong drugs, because if I went into a deep depression, I might decide that the pills would be the easy way out for me. I prayed to God that never happened.

I had been thinking quite a bit about my neck pain versus my back pain. I really believed that the intensity of pain I've felt dealt with my neck. My neck was more painful than my back. I don't know why, but that was the way I felt. I don't know if it was because of the headaches I also used to get when my neck hurt or not. I never used to get headaches at all before this injury. There is only one time I remember having a headache, and it was a bad one at that. I was home with Connie and my head began to hurt. With the kids around the neighborhood making noise and noise in the house, I went to my mother's house to lie down in my old bedroom. I stayed there all night, and when I woke up in the morning, the headache was gone. That was the first and last headache I remembered having.

Many times I think of other people who are going through all I have been through today. I wonder if they are feeling the same things which I am feeling. Are they suffering the same way I have over the last four months? What is their marriage is like compared to mine? Are they on a couch all the time like I am? Can they walk for a long period of time? I kind of wish I could find a group of people who are going through back pain today. It would also be nice if Connie could talk with someone. We both need to talk to someone very badly. The question is if we will really ever look for a group? I doubt it. Life will go on as it has in the past.

Many times, I would just lie back and think about all that Connie and I had been through. Our daughter Jen is our life. I always hoped that everything turned out much better for her than it did for us. I never even considered that I might end up getting hurt and our lives would end up in total chaos. I wish that things could have been better for us, but I am sure there is a reason why we have gone through all these problems. There are reasons for everything in life but, why this?

CHAPTER 15

I knew that I had to start thinking positive. Thinking about all the negatives only led to a depression. I had to continue thinking of the poor soldiers fighting these wars for us. They ended up being killed, hurt badly, and who knows what else. The things I was going through were a drop in the bucket compared to what they go through. Yes, I lived with pain every day, but I just couldn't dwell on it all the time. After all, my life could be much worse. When I had my back surgery, I was confident that I would feel great again. I just had to remember this.

I felt good going to the nursing home, but I was a little down, as many of these poor people were on their last trip before the big day came and they took the trip to heaven. So many people were happy to see someone like me. I truly realized that many of these people had no one to go and see them. They must be so lonely, and I hope that I don't end my life being lonely.

I went to the nursing home three more times before I realized that it was dragging me down. I loved all of the people I came into contact with, but I realized that I would not be going over there much longer. I wondered what these people would do when I stopped. I felt that they kind of looked forward to seeing me show up there, and when I stopped, it could be a letdown. That wasn't the reason I decided to begin visiting. I wish that I had thought things out more before I decided to go see these people.

I had an exceptionally busy month for November 2001. I was scheduled for physical therapy twelve times, along with seeing my doctor four times and having an x-ray of my back taken for Dr. Z. I hoped the time was coming. I really needed to have my back surgery. The pain was awful, and the lives Connie and I had been leading were almost nothing. We hadn't done anything for ourselves in a long time. I tried to see my mother as much as I could. I didn't have many visitors come to see me. Why, I didn't know.

I tried to not think about the place I had worked, because, in essence, I lost my life there. Very few people from my workplace had come to see me. I did have a couple of good friends who I helped get jobs there. I could always depend on them. I had to stop thinking about my old job, as it made me depressed, and I was already continually fighting depression. How could I be positive with all of the things that had happened to Connie and me? The thing that would turn me around was my back surgery. I knew I would feel good once again.

I continued to go to all of the appointments I had. Many times, I just wanted to stay home and say the hell with it, but I knew that I couldn't, as I had been through so much. I wasn't about to quit. So, I was up and ready to go to physical therapy and see all of the necessary doctors. The appointments I didn't mind were with Dr. Z, as he was the doctor who was going to put me back together.

Another problem I'd been having for quite some time was constipation. With all the drugs I was taking, I had an awful time going to the bathroom. At one point, I ended up in the hospital in Batavia for constipation, and the pain was unbearable.

We take so much for granted in our lives until the day comes when the pain follows the problem. When I fell, I hurt the sensation that we all have to warn us when it is time to go to the bathroom. My way of detecting this is to push on my stomach or realize that I have a bloated stomach. Granted, this is not a really effective way to realize that you need to have a BM, but this is the only way for me.

Each day, it seemed that something new came up that I really wasn't aware of with my body. It was often something small, but it was something that had changed my way of life. My sleeping habits became worse to where I never got a good night's sleep. I used to go to bed and sleep right through to the morning, but I found that I was now up a couple of times in the night and really didn't know why. Sometimes I had to urinate, but most of the time I didn't.

I was faced with taking things that made me go to the bathroom on a regular basis. Without the medication, I experienced a lot of pain in the stomach and back area, which was on top of the back pain I already had. Oh well, there are a lot of people who are much worse than me. I often had to remind myself that I should be happy that nothing worse had happened to me.

I hoped that after my back surgery, I would be back to my old self. There was no reason I shouldn't. When I had my first back surgery, it turned out great, and I felt the best I had in years. I was looking forward to that day again.

The time in my life seemed to move very slowly. I had many physical therapy sessions, along with my psychiatrist and psychologist visits. In between these appointments, I had my neurosurgeon and pain specialist to see weekly. Then I had to have MRIs, CAT scans, and anything else necessary to determine what had changed in my neck. I was beginning to pray on a regular basis to my God to get my life back again. I had suffered with this pain way to long.

CHAPTER 16

Starting in the beginning of 2002, I was also dealing with lawyers, workman's compensation, and social security disability. Connie and I were on the move all of the time. I am very glad she was able to stay home with me, as I know that I would not have been able to handle everything on my own. However, I also realized that we were losing a lot of money that she could be making, but this was the only way we could deal with all of this.

In February, we finally decided to go to Batavia to get a bed for me. The couch had worked okay, but I needed a bed to sleep on. I had no idea what kind of bed I was going to buy. We drove to Batavia on a Saturday morning and stopped off at the place where I'd bought the water beds. The man I bought the other beds from was there, and I told him about my back problem. Almost right away, he suggested an air bed.

I had never thought of an air bed before, but while lying down on one, I had so much comfort. There was also a controller to adjust the amount of air in the bed. This would depend on how bad or how good my back was at the time. After spending about an hour talking about the air bed, I decided to buy one. The bed was to be delivered on Monday afternoon. It worked out great, and Connie had the couch back again. The only problem was I'd really made a mess out of it, so I could see we would have to buy a new living room suite.

My neurosurgeon wanted me to be fitted for a back brace to see if it improved the pain I was having. This happened to be the first of two braces for which I was fitted over a period of six months. The brace, I could tell, was going to be very expensive, as it was going to work on the premise of a pump and air. I would place the brace around my stomach area and use the pump to increase the air pressure, which would supposedly relieve the pain in my back. After wearing this for about two months, I stopped using it, primarily because I couldn't sit down with it.

Well, I had now tried two braces for my back, and neither one worked. I just wondered what was going to happen next.

On March 27, 2002, I woke up with very bad chest pains and was rushed to the hospital via ambulance. After being tested for two days, they did find a spot on my lung but decided it was something that was not going to give me any problems. We would revisit the spot each year. I was released from the hospital on March 29 and returned home. Things were the same with pain, and everything continued looking up until the middle of April when I had another problem.

On April 14, 2002, I was rushed to the hospital with awful pain in my stomach area. I ended up having gall bladder surgery on April 17. There was a problem, as I had a lot of scar tissue from an old operation. They would have to open my stomach completely up instead of the short surgery that was available. I was in the hospital six days and then was allowed to come home. A few days after getting home, I had to go to Rochester to see my heart doctor. I didn't know what was going on, but everyone wanted to see me all of a sudden.

I began getting depositions from the attorneys about the accident, and I really worried that things might be going too quickly. I knew nothing about lawsuits, but a couple of my friends told me it looked like the people which I was suing wanted to get this over with. I guess I had to put my faith in my attorneys. I hoped that strategy didn't blow up in my face in the end.

From May through December, my psychiatrist visits began to increase, as I was still having a lot of pain, and it seemed like my surgeon might not be operating. The pain was as bad as it had ever been in my back, but the doctors were trying all these different things to see if they helped. I didn't mind trying things out, but Dr. Z had already told me that he needed to operate. I didn't know what the problem was.

During my next visit with Dr. L, I really came apart. I didn't know what to do, and I was really becoming depressed. I really thought I might be able to go back to work, but I had started questioning as to whether I would. I was not ready to stop working yet. I had enjoyed what I was doing, and I knew that I had nothing to really keep me busy if I did. On top of that, the insurance would be so expensive, and I would need to have a lot of money in order to pay all of the bills. We had investments, but we needed them for later in life.

I had not called my mother in a while and got very anxious to see her. I knew that I wasn't going to see her for a while, as she had moved in with my sister Sharon since Rozella's passing. I needed to see my mom. I didn't know what to do, but I had to do something. I was talking to my sister Sharon about seeing her, and she told me about this device that attached to the telephone. When you placed a call, there was a small screen that you could use to view the party that was on the receiving end of the phone. This sounded great, and I had to check into it.

I had been so close to my mother for many years. Ever since I was sick early in my life, we have been very close. I would see her regularly or call her almost every day. Well, now that I couldn't see her, it bothered me very much.

I had started to feel a little better then and not as depressed as I had been. If I could get to the point of talking with my mother, I knew it would help me greatly. Connie had also been so good to me. She'd done everything for me, even when she didn't feel well. The pain she had been living with over the years had really created many problems for her. She'd never really complained. Unfortunately, all of her family members had passed on. She really had no one close in her family to talk to. She was an only child, and her dad died in 1959 and her mom in 1980.

Connie had a couple of close friends, but one had cancer and wasn't expected to live. Connie had been very close to Diane for many years, as

Diane had been to us. Diane's husband, David, had been to our house many times to help out when we had a problem. When you have a bad back, you can't do anything, and David had been a very big help. So Connie had one good friend left who was close and was raising a child. So, basically, Connie was alone other than Jen and me.

I had undergone more MRIs and CAT scans, along with the regular doctors' appointments, and still nothing with my back operation.

With the information Sharon gave me about the video attachment to the phone, I got on the computer to search for such a device. I found a video monitor that did exactly what Sharon had told me. It was made by Vialta, and it attached to a standard home phone. There had to be two units one at my house and one at my sister Sharon's house in Connecticut. After hooking it up to both phones per the instructions, the caller would dial the number, and the recipient would pick the phone up. Each would then push a button, and then both the caller and the recipient could see each other through the TV screens. This new gadget worked just great, and I would call my mother each day and see her. My life was completely changed with this new device. I couldn't help but think, *Thank you, God, for all your help.*

I was so happy to be able to see my mom every day. She is so special to me, and being able to see her had definitely helped my depression.

CHAPTER 17

At the end of April, all of my physical therapy sessions had stopped. I had been through everything the pain specialist had wanted me to go through. After the gall bladder surgery, I had to take it easy for a couple of weeks before I tried to do anything.

I had been thinking a lot lately about the life Connie and I no longer had. There were so many things we were missing out on. I had robbed my wife of total happiness because of my injury. I didn't blame myself for falling, but I did blame myself for all of the things that had happened since being hurt. The love that we once shared together had been gone since my fall. I had a funny feeling in my back with different things that were normal, everyday happenings. When I had a BM, I couldn't determine when I had gone. I had the same problem with urination. I knew that I had damaged some nerves in my spinal cord badly.

The love life Connie and I shared had completely left us by this point. I didn't know if there would ever be another chance for me to make love to my beautiful wife, but there was nothing I could do about it.

There were many things that went through my mind daily. I continued to think about death on a regular basis. I had talked with Dr. Le about this, and he reconfirmed that when a person has a devastating accident, the patient might think about this on a fairly regular basis. These thoughts really bothered me, but there was nothing I could do.

Why couldn't people understand what I had been going through? Unfortunately, no one can know unless it happens to him. Not even Connie understood what I was going through. She couldn't understand how I could feel pretty good one minute and the next feel really bad.

I once found a letter about a person who was in the same situation as me. The letter described our lives perfectly. It was a letter to the "normals." This is what was so hard on me. Connie sometimes forgot the pain I was going through. I knew that she had her own pain, and I tried to sympathize with her. But when the shoe is on the other foot, she cannot understand. Maybe I cried wolf a lot, but I really didn't think so. The pain was there all of the time, and I had very little brake from it. Only when I lie down do I feel a little better. I wished that there were a way for me to show Connie what pain I was going through, but there wasn't.

I hoped that when I went to court I would be awarded a very reasonable amount of money for what I have been through. But I feared this would not happen, as no one could understand the hell that a person like me goes through. I really hoped that I can get better after my back surgery, as life with this pain was so bad. Even though I knew I was lucky for not dying, it still had created a hell I lived with every minute of every day. At times, I didn't care whether I lived or died. I often wondered what was left for me if I remained the way I was for the rest of my life.

I would promise one thing when I got better—if I got better. I would do anything I could to help other people with pain. It is so debilitating to a person. It makes it even harder when there is no compassion for that individual who is fighting every day just to feel a little bit better. This subject is so big, and as I said before, unless you have been through something like this, no one, and I mean no one, can even imagine how bad it gets. I know that when people commit suicide because of pain, it is hard for someone to understand why. Ask me, and I will tell you.

CHAPTER 18

In May 2002, I had to face a deposition, along with a workman's compensation hearing. The deposition had to do with the lawsuit for my fall. I had to face a lawyer from the person I was suing, along with my lawyer, and tell them both what happened. The timing of this was not good because of all the pain I was living with in my back. I didn't understand why the lawsuit had been started as soon given that not everything had been done yet, but I am not a lawyer. I just hoped that I didn't get screwed in all of this. It did not feel good at that point. I really thought we were moving ahead too quickly, but I had to follow what they said. Because of my back, I had not been to my back therapy in quite a while.

After the hearing, I would be off a week with nothing to do, and then the week of the twelfth I had to see the neurosurgeon, psychologist, and Dr. Le, whom I am looking forward to seeing. I had so much to talk about, as I was really having a hard time handling everything again. I had no one to talk to at home about the problems I was facing. I was trying to be strong for my wife and handle the normal, everyday activities, but that was no longer possible for me. Connie had to handle almost everything in the house, and that hurt me. I kept wondering if it would ever get better.

My prayers to God continued daily, and I don't think that I had ever received any answers up to that point. I remember praying: *How much can we withstand? Why are we going through all of this hell with no relief in sight? We are being punished severely for something that has happened in our lives. It's not fair. It's not fair. Let me suffer and give Connie some glimmer of hope to what is happening to us. I will bear the brunt of the load of pain and despair, but please lighten up on my beautiful wife. Take me, God, if you want me. I will be ready to go any time, but leave my wife alone. She has gone through so much in her life and now me.*

The days passed, and I was finally ready to see Dr. Le. I had thought of so many things to talk to him about, and I hoped I wouldn't forget to cover them all. We got to the building and went in the front door. I then signed in, and Connie sat down while I paced. Soon, Dr. Le said hello to us both and then invited me in.

As I walked through the door, I broke down right away. I told him that I could not handle all of this anymore. I told him I didn't care whether I lived or died. Quietly, he said to me, "Do you feel that you should be put into the hospital again?" My comment to him was no, but it was just all piling up on us—the pain in my back and not knowing about the back surgery. There were no positive things happening to us anymore. He had told me that things would get better, but I had to be a little more patient. He then suggested that we see each other the following week, which was not normal, but he wanted to see me again.

We talked for an hour, and he increased the medication I had for despair. I did feel much better when I left, and I had the appointment set for the following week. The talks that we had always got to the point of the problem. The psychiatrists I had seen in the past were always hurrying to get me out of there. I never felt that they cared about my problems. But Dr. Le had always been very concerned about me, and I cared for him a lot because of this. I felt at ease seeing him, and it had helped me a lot.

The last week of the month found me with my neurosurgeon again. He continued to order a new MRI every couple of months so he could keep comparing the condition of my back. I kept asking him when or if he was going to operate on my back. He continued to tell me that it was not time yet. He had to make sure he knew what was happening. I really didn't know what he meant, but I supposed that I had to continue to be patient while I was suffering.

By June 2002, I had no guesses as to how long I was going to continue to suffer. It had dragged on so long that I figured I would be like this for the rest of my life. I had been so down because there had been funny comments about the pain I lived with. At times, I could feel pretty good and then ten minutes later feel like hell. I didn't know why that happened, but it was very normal with me. In fact, it had happened so many times that Connie had questioned me on this.

People who have lived with very bad pain for a long period of time know what I am talking about. Connie said to me quite a few times that she couldn't understand how things could change so quickly. I wish I knew the answer, but I don't. I live through hell each day of my life.

I had developed a bad tooth problem and was very concerned about trying to sit in the dentist's chair. I was really worried, but the pain in my tooth was very bad. I thought about it for about a minute, and then Connie made an appointment for me with the dentist. I was fortunate that he could see me the next day. The pain in my tooth almost overrode the pain in my back.

I tried to lie down on the couch, hoping that the pain in my mouth would lighten up. How stupid I was to think that? Nothing changed at all. The pain became very intense in my mouth. I began to get a very bad headache, which I hated. There were no pain pills I could take, as I was already taking some highly potent stuff.

As I lay on my bed, I gradually fell asleep. I sure as hell don't know how I did, but it happened. I only slept for about two hours, but when I awoke, I felt a little bit better. As I began to get up, Connie suggested that I use some tooth medication she had in the medicine cabinet. I couldn't get it on quick enough, and I was pleased that it definitely worked. It didn't last a long time, but it was long enough to give me relief.

I decided to go to bed early that night. I knew I'd just woken up a couple of hours earlier and it was only nine thirty, but I was really tired. So, I went to bed and soon feel a sleep. I was up a few times in the night going to the bathroom and dealing with the tooth problem, but before I knew it, seven thirty had arrived on my clock. I got up to get a drink and then decided to lie down again for another hour. I got Connie up, as my appointment with the dentist was at eleven thirty. It was at that point when I began worrying about sitting in the dentist's chair. I did have some Hydrocodone, which I would take an hour before we left.

We got ready after Connie got up, and I popped a Hydrocodone at ten thirty. We drove to the dentist, and I was really beginning to worry. We pulled into the parking lot and got out of the car. We went in and were greeted by the dentist's staff. We waited about ten minutes before I was called in. The dentist was very compassionate toward my back problem and really took his time doing everything. I had brought a pillow we had at home to sit on that would hopefully make my back feel a little better while I was in the chair.

As I lowered myself onto the chair, the pain began to rush to my head and brain. When I finally sat down all the way, it was painful but not as bad as I thought it might be. I was sure it was because I had taken that Hydrocodone earlier. The doctor located my problem tooth after I pointed it out to him.

It turned out that I had a small cavity, which evidently had loosened the old filling and exposed my nerve. He explained the situation and then proceeded to fix the problem. I had made it through what I was so afraid of. I felt like a million dollars with respect to the tooth. However, my back still hurt, and I was sure I was going to pay for it when I stood up.

The moment of reckoning had come. The dentist moved the chair slowly to where I could get up. As I began to stand, I again felt the pain rush to my head. I began to get very nervous, as I expected a very bad headache like I'd had just a day earlier. Fortunately, the headache never came, but the pain in my back was astounding. As I got out of the chair, I crippled up the worst I'd ever had. I had to walk like a one hundred-year-old man, all slumped over. Both the dentist and I couldn't believe how slouched over I was. He immediately asked me if I was all right. I told him I was but added that I couldn't straighten right away. I assured him not to worry, as

I would be better after I walked awhile. He made sure to watch me until my back had loosened up so I could straighten up a bit more. I thanked the dentist for fitting me in, and he told me he was happy he could help me.

I got into the car very carefully, and Connie was really concerned that I was okay. I assured her that I was, but I really did hurt much more than I had before my appointment. As we were riding home, Connie did all she could to avoid the big bumps. We finally made it to our house, and I really took my time getting out of the car. When I did, I was again all crippled up as I'd been at the dentist's office. Getting out of the car was very painful, but I made it. At least I didn't have any tooth pain any longer.

I got into the house and immediately went to my bed. The pain in my back was as bad as it had ever been, but it was worth it to stop the tooth pain. As I lay there, Connie came up to me and gave me a little peck. I hoped that it was because she was proud of me for getting the problem taken care of. I finally drifted off to sleep and stayed there for about three hours. I woke up fairly hungry, as I had not eaten yet. Connie made me some soup, as I had to be careful of the new filling.

I took it easy for the rest of the day, and Connie decided that she was going to go out and do some shopping for groceries. I knew that she also wanted to get out of the house, as she hadn't been out by herself in quite some time. When she left, I watched TV while lying down. I again fell asleep for another two hours, and she walked in the house just as I was getting up. She knew that I had just woken up but said nothing to me. The rest of the night was laid back with both of us relaxing. I had been relaxing all day since we'd gotten home from the dentist. I got ready for bed at eleven and went to lie down after a kiss for my girl.

I woke up at eight the next morning. I had another meeting with Dr. Le that day. A week had already gone by, and it was time to see the doctor who had helped me so much. I woke Connie up at nine o'clock, as our appointment was at two. We had breakfast and took it easy for a while before getting ready. We showered and were ready to leave at one thirty. I got into the car first and then Connie, and we were off down the road.

We arrived at the office shortly before two o'clock went inside. My doctor was waiting as we walked in. I went into his office with him and took my normal position on his couch. He asked me how things were going compared to the previous week. I told him that things were much better. He asked me what I thought made me feel that way. I told him that maybe because a couple of good things had happened to us. He was happy for me.

We talked for an hour, and the session was over. He told me he would see me in a couple of weeks if it was okay. I told him yes, and then Connie and I left. I told Connie I had a much better meeting with Dr. Le, and she was happy for me.

A few days later, I had to see Dr. Z again. I had to have some MRIs done, which I did, and we had the results to bring with us. The time went by quickly until our meeting with Dr. Z. We went into the office with the MRI results and sat in the huge waiting area to be called. We had signed in, and Connie sat while I paced, as usual. We then were called for our meeting with the doctor. We greeted him as we walked in.

I handed the MRI results to him, and he reviewed the information. He evidently had seen something there that had changed, as he told me that he didn't want me to have any more physical therapy for now. I asked the reason, and he told me that therapy was not working, so there was no reason to continue it. This news kind of made me happy. I was going so much that I really hurt much more when I got home. I would prefer to devote my time to the doctors' appointments.

Dr. Z and I stayed another ten minutes and then left. He had given me another appointment for two weeks again.

I really thought that he'd seen something and just didn't want to alarm us. I knew there was a problem with my back from all the pain I was having. This was the same situation as with my neck.

CHAPTER 19

I fell in October 2000 and finally received an operation in August 2001, which was almost a year later. This bothered me very much. I wondered what was holding everything up, but, of course, I am not the doctor. Oh how I wished that the pain I lived with day and night would stop. My mind was so confused, and I really didn't think that I want to continue like this any longer. Connie would definitely be better off without me. I had to get the thoughts out of my head. All I would do would be to create more problems for Connie.

We got through the month of May with everything remaining the same. I had seen my neurosurgeon three times during the month, along with my psychiatrist. I made the decision that I was not going to cry around anymore, as I had already done. I could see that Connie was also really getting depressed about how the way I feel.

Connie's birthday was on June 17, and I was going to try to give her a nice day. I planned to get a cake and asked some of the neighbors over for cake and ice cream. I hoped that Connie had a good time. Unfortunately, Jen had to work, so she wouldn't be able to stop by. I decided to get a gift card for Connie and give her some perfume or something like that.

But first, I had to have some more MRIs, along with going back to the dentist. The MRIs were all of my back, and I couldn't believe that I'd had four of these in the past couple of months. I could tell that the doctor really saw something, but he wasn't saying what it was. I had asked him quite a few times what the problem was, but he had not said anything to me. Hopefully, I could have this operation soon, as it really was eating me up inside.

I often found myself wondering what had happened to me. So many things had changed since I'd been hurt at work. The pain I have gone through has been the worst I have ever had. With all of the medication I took, urinating and having BMs had been very difficult for me. To not have the normal sense of knowing when I have to go to the bathroom really creates something very different for me. I can't believe that I have to push on my stomach in order to go to the bathroom. I wondered what other damage I created by falling down those stairs.

I was also having a very rough time with the gas in my stomach. I experienced huge buildups of gas after drinking soda. I always used to get rid of the gas with no problems. Now, I often get to be really bloated and also have to go into the bathroom to push on my stomach so it will move the gas around and enable me to release it. The tightness of my under shorts where my band is, can be so sensitive that I have to remove them every night.

Sleeping on my bed had been great, and I really enjoyed lying down now. My sleep had been very poor, and I was not getting a good, quality sleep. Thank God I felt better when I went to lie down. I don't know what I would do if I had the awful pain all night long.

Connie had been a very big help to me by trying to get me to lose weight, which I realized may help a lot. However, I had not gotten to the point where I'd lost a lot of weight. I realized that this was something I had to do.

The devices I've had to be fitted for that were designed to give me some sense of relief did not work like I thought they might. I was really hoping they would work so I could cut down on my pain medication, which, in turn, would resolve the problems I had with going to the bathroom.

At one point, I began taking quite a bit of milk of magnesia, as the pain from trying to go to the bathroom was fairly intense. Connie also developed a special mixture of applesauce, prune juice, and bran flakes that she chilled in the refrigerator overnight. I then took about four tablespoons in the morning and at night. The idea was the concoction would make me loose enough that I could go without really straining.

I began to pray more often that I would be able to have surgery on my back soon. I felt as though I couldn't hold out to much longer. I tried to sit down with a close friend of mine about all the pain and what it was doing to me mentally. It has really scared me the last few weeks as I cannot handle this pain to much longer. The toll it was taking and the thought of what I may do to stop the awful pain really scared me. I really feel bad for all of those servicemen who are committing suicide today, but what was I going to do?

My sister Sharon had stepped up since Rozella passed away and was a very big help to me. Sharon had been a very big piece of my life and helped me to get through all of this.

There came I time when I began looking information up on the computer about falls and back surgeries. I was trying to find out anything I could to determine what might be wrong with me. Even though I was going through all of this pain, I still need to find what Dr. Z may be looking at. I didn't know what the results may be when determining what type of surgery he would perform—if he performed surgery at all.

I found that there are many operations that are performed on the back every day, but doctors don't like to operate if they don't have to. The reason for this is because of failed back surgeries, which are never actually the best for the patient. I sure hoped that Dr. Z would make the correct move for me. After all, this was my life we were talking about.

I also tried to talk with people I might know who have had back problems. One person I really knew, and who happened to be one of the owners of our company, has since passed away. At one time, he told me he had eight back surgeries and still didn't feel really good. This is what the books talk about regarding doctors who are afraid to operate on a patient's back, as it turns out to be a flip of a coin. I don't know what I would do if I was operated on and my back still hurt afterward. I decided that I would have to really think about whether I wanted to take the chance on surgery. But

I couldn't help but wonder what else I would do. The pain I was living with was just awful. So many times I couldn't even think because the pain was so bad.

I remember my dad telling me years ago that he'd broken his back when his old Model T turned over. At that time, there were no x-rays or any other type of test to determine what the problem was or how bad it was. He used to come home from work when I was still in high school, and he would have to lie on the floor so I could rub his back. The pain he went through was just awful. One time I suggested that we put Absorbine on his back. This was a liniment that our basketball coach used on our knees and backs when they hurt. It was a very strong liquid, which was used on horses' legs for swelling. As my dad lay on the rug, I put some on, and it sipped down his crack. He got up screaming and ran around the house in pain. At the time, we laughed, but it was no laughing matter. Finally, in the mid-1950s, he had an x-ray and found his back was broken.

My dad would have been a wealth of information about pain, but unfortunately, he passed away in 1985. He was such a strong person. He very rarely complained about his health even though he was going through hell. If I would have been half the man he was, I would be a martyr.

CHAPTER 20

By November, I'd had many appointments. Between my head doctors and therapy sessions when I could, I was on the move all the time. I really felt that this time that I was getting closer to having surgery. I was very convinced that I was going to have the surgery, as the pain had been awful, and I couldn't stand it much longer. Even though it was taking a big chance, I had to go for it. What was the worst that could happen? The worst was that I'd end up in a lot more pain than I already had, which I doubted would happen. I prayed to God that everything would turn out all right when I had the surgery. I saw all my doctors and had all of the necessary tests for the month.

My appointment with Dr. Z was on December 4. Connie and I got there early, and I really hoped that this would be the day he told me he would operate. He walked into the room, greeted us, and asked me how I was feeling. I told him lousy. He said that was good, as he was going to operate on January 14, 2003. I began to cry. It had been almost three years since my fall, and I was finally going to have the surgery. I actually went up and hugged Dr. Z. I was so happy. He told us to call the office next week to get the information.

Connie and I drove home from his office. I was so happy that the time was finally here. I couldn't wait to let everyone know. When we got home, I couldn't wait to call my family. I called Jen and then my mom and sisters. I was thrilled, and I thanked God for stepping in to get it done. I still couldn't believe it. I was so damn happy.

Hopefully, this would result in no more pain, or at least less pain. After I made the calls, I realized how bad my back felt from the ride. I'd forgotten about the pain because of the good news. I had to lie down and get off of my feet. As soon as I hit the pillow, I went right to sleep. I had more than a month before my surgery.

When I woke up, I was still very happy and excited. I had suffered long enough and hoped all would be better soon. I grabbed Connie and gave her a big kiss. The night went fairly slowly, and I watched TV with Connie. When it was ten thirty, I decided to go to sleep. After getting ready, I went to lie on the bed and gradually fell asleep. I woke up at eight o'clock the next morning. I had to go to physical therapy, and it would be my last day. *Thank God*, I thought, as I'd had enough of this. The surgery would straighten everything out. The therapist congratulated me and wished me luck with the surgery.

I had an appointment with my psychiatrist the following afternoon. The rest of the day went quickly, and I received some phone calls from friends who had heard I was going to have my surgery.

I went to bed early and was up at seven o'clock in the morning. I had gotten Connie up at nine, and we started to get ready at about ten thirty. We got in the car at one thirty and arrived at Dr. L's office just before two o'clock.

When I went back for my appointment, I told him of my good fortune, and he was very happy for me. I lay down, and we had a good talk. He asked me how I felt. I told him that I had not been so happy since before I'd fallen. He asked me if I had any worries about the surgery. I told him the only thing I was worried about was the possibility that the surgery wouldn't be a success.

He then asked me how I would handle it if my surgery wasn't a success. I told him one day at a time. We talked for an hour, and when I was ready to leave, I hugged him. I really felt that he had helped me keep my act together and had saved me a couple of times when I was thinking about doing some bad things to myself. He wanted to see me again after the surgery. We scheduled an appointment on March 15, which was two months after the surgery. I thanked him and left.

Connie and I got in the car and drove back to Le Roy. She had to call Dr. Z's office to get the info regarding the surgery. When we got home, I went to lie down for a short time. Connie had decided to call after having a cigarette. She soon made the call and got all the information. We would talk about it the next day, as she had some things she had to finish before the end of the day.

I decided to see if I could do a few things around the house to help Connie. There were dishes in the dishwasher that I dried off for her. I hadn't done that in a long time. It felt good to help, but my back was really hurting from bending over. I then went into my bedroom and used the vacum cleaner. Using the cleaner really hurt my back, and I really don't know why I did it other than I felt it was time to start helping her more. I was now done and would do no more for the day.

We had dinner and then watched TV in the evening. I decided to go to bed at ten. I got ready for bed, kissed Connie, and went to bed. I soon fell asleep. I was up a couple of times during the night and finally woke up at eight o'clock the next morning. Connie got up at ten. She sat around for a while and then got dressed. We discussed the information she'd received from Dr. Z's office and would go over it again just before the day I was to be operated on.

I had no appointments on that day, but the following day I had two doctors' visits in Batavia. I also had an appointment with the lawyer that week to talk about my lawsuit. The pain I had was still there, but I had been trying to block it out of my mind.

I thought a lot about my surgery that week. To get my life back would be so great. I had so many things I wanted to do. Maybe I could even go back to work, which would be great. I imagined what it would be like to get back with people again and be busy during the day. I prayed to my God above that I could feel good again. It has been almost two and a half years since I had worked. It would be so nice to work again.

I realized that I needed to stop thinking about these things and get some things done. November was a slow month for us. There were no more therapy sessions and hopefully not many other doctor appointments other than Dr. Z. I did have a CAT scan scheduled for December 10 and then an appointment on December 19 for the fitting of my back brace, which I would have to wear after my surgery.

I hadn't even done any Christmas shopping yet. I didn't know what Connie wanted for Christmas. I figured I would get her some perfume and a one-hundred-dollar gift certificate to JCPenney. I knew it was going to be a very different Christmas than the year before, but a year earlier there wasn't much to be happy about. This year was much different.

My Christmas present was going to be my surgery in January. That's all I wanted for Christmas. I couldn't help but think about all the things I was going to be able to do again. It would be just like the surgery I had in 1986. I'd felt great after that surgery was over with. I couldn't wait for my upcoming surgery. *Thank you, God,* I thought, *for all that you have done for me.*

I had the CAT scan done and then went and had the fitting for my new back brace. The back brace was fairly large and made of very heavy plastic. The individual measured my chest and around my waste. The brace would be done in a week, and we had to pick it up about December 27.

It was now the twenty-first, and Connie was going to Rochester to shop for the afternoon. I decided to get into my car and drive to Crocker's Ace Hardware to see my friends there. I stopped for about twenty minutes and went back home. My back was bothering me quite a bit, so I decided to lie down and watch TV. After lying down, I fell to sleep very quickly and slept for about three hours. When I woke up, I remembered that we had nothing out for dinner, so I pulled some hot dogs out of the freezer and put them into a pan with hot water to thaw out. Fortunately, we had some hot dog buns, and with chips, we would have a good dinner.

Connie came home about five thirty with bags of Christmas gifts. She told me not to look at a couple of bags she brought in and set on the Christmas table. I stayed away from the two bags and helped her with the others by taking them to her bedroom. She had gotten all of her shopping done, as had I. I hoped that this would be a better Christmas than it had been the year before.

I had no more appointments for the balance of December. We both had our shopping done, and all I had to do was a little wrapping. I knew that she also had to wrap, so I helped her with that.

My pain was quite bad that day, and my back ached so badly. I had worked around the day before to help Connie, and I knew that this would happen. Oh well, I enjoyed doing things when I could. I often knew that the outcome was going to be suffering—that was just life.

Jen did all she could to help us, but she had problems of her own. I was so proud of our little girl, who had grown up to be such a beautiful person. Adopting her was the very best thing that ever happened to Connie and me. She went through school as a good student and always worked hard at whatever she did. She was going to go far in life. We were so happy that she had accepted us the way she had.

CHAPTER 21

It was Christmas morning in the United States. Unfortunately, Connie and I had decided not to put up a Christmas tree. Connie just didn't want to have it, and I didn't care. Our Christmases since Jen had left were not the nice days they had been. Jen would be coming to dinner that night, and we couldn't wait to see her. Since she had gotten married again and began working at Strong, we saw her very little. But we would see her that night. Our baby would be with us on Christmas.

Jen came to dinner and brought some small gifts with her. We didn't care about any gifts but enjoyed getting her nice things. She didn't make a lot of money, so her gifts to us were small, and that was fine with us. Her eyes lit up so bright when she opened something that she may have told Connie she wanted. Our Jen is just a great daughter.

Connie made a nice meal, and Jen stuck around for a couple of hours and then had to go. Our Christmas was over. Jenny was our Christmas. I gave Connie the couple of gifts I'd gotten her, and she gave me a couple of things. We kissed each other and cried together; we loved each other so much.

CHAPTER 22

Lately, I had been having some problems getting my patches. Rite Aid Pharmacy had been having problems getting the correct patches in stock. I'd already had to go to different pharmacies to pick up my correct patches a couple of different times. Just as long as I was able to keep getting the right ones, I had no problem. But the day that a problem did occur, I would find a different drug store to deal with.

I had a pre-op appointment the following day at the hospital. I needed to be there at twelve fifteen. My back had been giving me trouble again. Once again, I'd done a couple of things around the house that I shouldn't have, and now I was paying for it. I wanted to help as much as I could around the house. Connie hadn't been getting out lately, and I was trying to push her to get out and see some friends. She told me she just didn't care to. I just figured that one of these days she'd start to get out. After my surgery, she could go out and raise hell. We would be able to go out to eat again.

In just a few more days, I would have my surgery. Hopefully, the pain would become a thing of the past. My neck has progressed and was a lot better. My pain level was much better than it was prior to the neck surgery. I wouldn't have believed that my neck would feel as good as it did. I was so lucky to have such good doctors. My pain was much better, and I foresaw my life being as good as it was before I'd been hurt.

I began to think about all of the things I had missed out on in the past couple of years. Connie had to haul me all over, and I had to sleep on the couch. One of the big things aside from the pain was the mental problems

I had to go through. I was really going to enjoy my life again, and I knew I had a lot to make up to my beautiful wife and daughter.

I also wondered how quickly I would be able to go back to work. With all the crap we had gone through, I almost wanted to find another job and get out of the place that helped hurt us so bad. I did like it there, but they, in essence, had ruined part of my life. I would have to continue to think about that for a few more days before I decided.

My back was really hurting today which was January 12, 2003. I really hadn't done too much the day before, but my back was really beginning to hurt quite a bit. My surgery was going to be in two days, and I couldn't wait. Many people become so afraid when they hear the word *surgery*. I guess that I couldn't blame them, as I used to be the same way. But I'd had so many surgeries that it no longer bothered me.

I got through the day just taking it easy. I watched TV and spent the day lying around doing nothing. Connie ordered a pizza for dinner from our favorite pizza place and cheated with some wings too. After filling ourselves up, we watched TV for the rest of the night until eleven o'clock when I finally went to bed. I got up once during the night to go to the bathroom and then slept through until about seven thirty when I got off the couch. Connie slept in until nine o'clock and then was up for the day. The following day was surgery. I was really getting kind of excited, as all I could think about was getting back to the things I used to do.

I couldn't wait to cut the lawn and do things around the house again. Hopefully, I would have my life back again. I decided to think positive. I also decided to really take it easy that day. I was not going to take a chance that the surgery might have to be postponed because I had done something wrong. And so, I decided to lie down and watch TV for the day. I watched TV until dinnertime, and then we had to eat what was in the freezer. I didn't take anything out to eat, so we must eat out of the freezer. Connie didn't mind. We both picked what we wanted and then consumed it. We had to be at the hospital at seven thirty the following morning, so we had to be up by four thirty.

When we were done with dinner, I went to lie back down and watch TV. Before I knew it, ten thirty had rolled around, and I got ready for bed. I then gave Connie a kiss and slid off to sleep. I woke up about two thirty and had to go the bathroom. Then it was back to bed. At about quarter after four, I got up and put the coffeepot on. I woke Connie up at four thirty and then went in and took a quick shower. When I got done, Connie was ready, and then she got in the shower. She then got a little to eat; unfortunately, I could not eat anything.

This was the morning of January 14, 2003—the morning of my back surgery. I was ready.

We were getting in the car at six thirty to begin our drive to Rochester. I hadn't even really thought about the surgery too much. My back was about a seven on the pain scale, but I knew that when we got to Rochester and I stepped out of the car, my pain level will be a nine or ten.

We drove about forty-five minutes and pulled into the parking lot at the hospital. When I got out of the car, I was crippled up. My back really hurt very bad, and I again thought about after the surgery. After about ten minutes of walking, I felt much better. We then walked into the hospital.

We went to the insurance desk and checked in. It took about ten minutes, and then an aid with a wheelchair was there to wheel me to my room. We got on to the elevator and went to room number 305 on the third floor. This was the surgical floor. A nurse came in with a gown for me to put on and instructed me to give Connie any valuables. The nurse came back in about ten minutes to start an IV in my arm. After looking for a vein, she pulled the cap off of the needle and told me I would feel a little prick. Because I have had so many needles in my lifetime, there was very little pain at all. The IV was in, and I was ready to go.

The nurse got everything done that was needed, and then she left. Connie and I began talking when Dr. Z walked in with his surgical gown and hat on. He asked me if I had any questions and then told me that the surgery would take about five hours. He told me he would see me in the operating room and left. About ten minutes later, the anesthesiologist came in and explained a couple of things he would be doing. I thanked him, and he left. The nurse again came in the room and said that I would be leaving for surgery in five minutes. I gave Connie a kiss, and before I knew it, I was being wheeled out of the door to surgery. I told Connie I loved her, and she said the same to me.

When I got to the operating room, I was given a shot into my IV, which would put me to sleep. About five hours later, I woke up in the recovery room. I was still quite groggy but felt an awful pain coming from my back area. I also felt this big back brace, which was used to keep me from moving and hurting my back again. I would fade in and out and still was quite tired. After about an hour, I was taken to my room. Connie was there waiting for me, and I was still very groggy. My sister was also there with Connie, awaiting my return to the room. I began to feel the pain more and began moaning. After roughly half an hour, a nurse came in and gave me a pain shot. It was about fifteen to twenty minutes before the shot had taken effect in my bloodstream, and I then went to sleep.

Dr. Z had come to see Connie shortly after I got to the room. He told Connie that the surgery had gone well. He told her that he had to fuse my back L-2, L-2, L-3, L-4, L-5, S-1 and then had inserted two steel rods and a cage assembly. The doctor felt that I should be in much better shape with my back now that the surgery had been completed. I'd had quite a mess in my back after the fall. Connie was very happy that the surgery was over and that the doctor felt it was a success. He told Connie he would stop by again the following day to see me.

I was in and out for most of that afternoon and evening. When I could feel the area around my back, it was very painful. I thought that my back was normally bad, but this was really painful. I really hoped that Dr. Z's work would take care of all of the problems I had been having. My sister was very impressed at what the doctor said and really hoped that I would now feel much better.

I finally woke up at about ten o'clock that night, and Connie and my sister were still there. I was so glad to see them. I must have been dreaming, as I had remembered sometimes with my dad years ago. I was really confused and told Connie and my sister about the dream.

Because it was getting so late, the girls decided to go home together and leave a car in the hospital parking lot. They kissed me good-bye and left for the night.

During the night, I had a lot of pain. Aside from the surgery, the bed was really creating much more pain because the mattress was so firm. I was not used to sleeping on a mattress like this, and I really couldn't stand it with the surgery and my back. I asked for a pain shot a couple of times during the night. They finally woke me up at about seven o'clock in the morning so I could have breakfast. The phone rang at eight, and it was Connie calling to see how I was. After talking for about ten minutes, I lay back to feel the pain I had. I knew that it wouldn't last long, and I prayed that the result would be just great for me. I would be so happy.

A nurse walked in to tell me that we would be walking. Thinking about that really worried me, because I knew how bad it would be, and then I would have to return to this damn bed, which would absolutely kill me to lie on it after walking. *Oh well*, I thought. *I am tough!*

The nurse came in about an hour later and looked at me kind of funny, so I looked back at her kind of funny. All of a sudden, she said, "Walk time."

Oh shit, I thought, *here we go.*

The nurse helped me get up and turn to put my feet to the floor. But she all of a sudden stopped me and told me I needed slippers. I had none, so she used my shoes. I slid off the bed and onto my feet. At first, the pain just shot to my brain, but I knew I had to walk.

I finally had my feet on the floor. Then a second nurse came into the room to help steady me. I had one nurse on each arm. I felt real pain from my back, but I did put one foot ahead of the other and began walking down the hall. It took us about twenty minutes to walk twenty feet. I couldn't believe that, once again, I was walking just a few short hours after my surgery. I knew that I had to walk, but I'd forgotten how quickly that it had to be. When I got back to the room, I couldn't wait to lie down, as I was very tired.

The nurses told me that we would have to walk again in about three hours. So after lying down, I fell asleep. I must have slept for a couple of hours as I woke to a visitor.

A couple of friends from my old job had stopped by to see me. The lady was very concerned that they had come to see me too quickly. I told her it was okay. Just as we began talking again, Connie walked into the room and bent over to give me a kiss. She then said hello to our friends that had stopped by to see me. They said that they had to leave in a few minutes, as they had someplace to go. I thanked them for stopping by and asked them to stop again.

When they left, Connie asked how I was. I told her that the pain was not too bad, but I had just had a pain shot after we'd come back from my first walk. In fact, in about another thirty minutes, I would be taking my next walk.

Connie updated me on all that was happening home. She told me that several people had called to wish me well and would stop at the house when I got home. I told her that the pain I was feeling was from the surgery itself, but the two steel rods and cage they had put in my back was also very painful. I realized that I needed a cane to walk with for a while to keep my balance.

The next walk came and went. I had gone through three more days doing the same but increasing the length of the walk. I began to feel much better with my back pain, but it didn't feel as good as after the first surgery I'd had. *Oh well, I have to give it time*, I figured.

I was ready to go home on Friday, and it was great for me to finally get home. I was told I really had to take it easy and wear my back brace all of the time. The brace was really big, but it was necessary to protect my back.

When I had my first bowel movement after the surgery, something was very different, although I really didn't know what it was. The pain was awful, and the tears came flowing down my cheeks. It was awful pain, and I tried not to push. Thank God when I was done. It was so difficult for me to have a BM, and I realized that I was going to have to mention the problem to Dr. Z when I saw him again.

On Friday at two thirty, Connie had come after me to take me home. I couldn't wait to get home, and I bet they couldn't wait for me to leave. Connie put my back brace in the trunk, as I couldn't wear it in the car. I sat in the car seat and wondered what I was going to feel like when we got home.

After about fifty minutes, we pulled into the driveway. Getting out was very difficult, but I made it. I had to take my time to walk around first to get loosened up. When I got into the house, I immediately went to lie down. I was very tired and fell asleep right away.

I woke up about five thirty that evening. The phone had just rung, and Connie had picked it up. It was my mom wondering how I was. Connie had given me the phone, and I talked with my mom for about ten minutes. She then told me she would be over to see me the next day for a little while. I was really glad to talk with her, as I knew she was very worried about me going through this back surgery. But now I think she was really at ease. I was really looking forward to feeling much better so I could go back to work and do the things I enjoyed. I decided that I was going to go out and buy a cane to walk with. I still did not feel steady on my feet. If I didn't continue to get better, it looked like I may have to use the cane all of the time.

CHAPTER 23

About two weeks had gone by since my surgery, and I had an appointment to see Dr. Z to go over how I felt. Although I felt much better than I did, I still had pain in my neck and my back. Maybe this was normal for what I'd gone through. We would see. I also needed to discuss my bowel movements with the doctor.

Connie and I left at about twelve thirty to be there at one thirty. We got there, and both my back and neck hurt quite a bit after the ride. After I walked for a few minutes, we walked into the office. I went up and signed in, and then Connie sat down while I walked around.

After about ten minutes, we were called to go back to his office. He met us at the door and greeted us. We went in, and he asked me how I felt. I told him that my back and neck still hurt, and I had to use a cane, as I didn't feel steady on my feet. He began feeling around my back and neck and then said he wanted me to have another x-ray before I saw him again in a couple of weeks.

I asked him what he thought, but he just told us that he wanted to see the new x-rays before he said anything. He made an appointment for me to see him in two weeks. He still wanted me to do nothing but to walk at home until after I saw him again. I told him that the pain was hurting quite a bit but not as bad as before the surgery. Since I was already on the pain patch, he wasn't going to give me anything else. We left and drove home. The brace was very cumbersome, and I had to take it easy with it.

When we got home, I had to go through the same walk after I got out of the car. I then went in to lie down for a short time. I was much more tired than I originally thought when we got home. I had been in the hospital for four days and really had not been up a lot. I was going to have to take it easy, but I need the exercise to gain my strength back. After getting up, I was going to have to figure out where I was going to walk each day. I decided to would walk to a place about ten minutes from our house. This would be a good walk for me twice a day. I would start the next day. I had to remember the brace, though, and couldn't overdo it. I had to wear it every day, but thank God I didn't wear it when I went to bed.

The night went quickly, as I felt pretty good—much better than I had felt in a long time. This was great, and I appreciated it so much. I still had pain but not as bad as before my back surgery. I remembered that morning I'd forgotten to tell Dr. Z about my problems with the bowel movements.

I woke up at eight o'clock and looked forward to walking. I couldn't go anywhere in the car for a couple of weeks, so I had to keep busy. I would watch TV and walk and lie down. I did run into one very funny situation, but it wasn't funny at the time it happened.

I had walked outside around the house on one particular day. Then, a couple of hours later, I decided to take a walk to the cemetery. It wasn't a long walk, but in this case, it took longer than I expected. I began walking, and it was a beautiful day. I walked for about fifteen minutes until I got to the cemetery.

I had noticed after I got there that I was quite tired. I thought I would rest a few minutes and then head back home. So I just looked around and enjoyed the scenery. After about ten minutes, I decided to return to my house. As I started to leave, I realized that my legs were very tired. My legs would not move, and it appeared that I was stuck there at the cemetery. So I had to wait about twenty minutes until I was completely rested before I could go home. I learned a very big thing that day. The first was that I had to make sure if I went someplace I could get home. The next was to have a cell phone and to always have it with me.

I stayed away from the cemetery for a while after that, as I didn't want to have that problem again. Maybe I had walked too far for such a short time. I decided to stay on my street and only walk twice a day as I had been instructed.

At home, I tried to sit in a chair a couple of times, but I had quite a bit of pain so I stopped. The doctor told me I couldn't drive for at least a month, so I would be watching a lot of TV. Fortunately, I had some good friends, as they stopped by off and on to see how I was doing. One asked me if I was going back to work, and I kind of hollered and said, "Hell yes, I am going back to work." I needed to go back to work. I was too young to be retired because of a fall. Sure I hurt, but I had hurt before. I knew that this couldn't keep me down. I have experienced a lot of pain in my past. Thinking about it later on, after the person left, I really wondered if I would ever be able to go back to work again. I had two steel rods and a cage in my back and a steel plate in my neck. I really didn't know if I could come back from this. I sure hoped I could.

I took my walks each day. Physical therapy was out of the question for another month, and I didn't have any other doctors' appointments until mid-February. I had to go back to see my surgeon first, and I would then find out what I could or couldn't do.

The pain I had was being taken care of with the patch or even hydrocodone if the pain was too much. Things seemed to be going pretty well, but it was still hard to sleep. The pain from my stitches really hurt but not like the pain I had before the operation. I was doing okay, but we would see as time went on.

Another two weeks had passed, and I began building my strength up pretty well. I had to see my surgeon the next afternoon. I had quite a few questions I wanted to ask him. I didn't know if he would have the answers, but I hoped he would.

Connie and I watched TV for the evening and then went to bed a little early. I went to bed at ten o'clock, and Connie had stayed up a while later. We both were up at about seven o'clock the following morning and sat down for a cup of coffee. We took our time getting ready, and by noon, we were ready to get in the car and head for Rochester. I was not going to get negative until I was really sure. I had noticed some changes in my BMs and urination. I had mentioned this to the doctor, and he wanted me to have more x-rays in a few weeks to look at something in my back.

When we got home, the pain I had was rough. I slid off the front seat of the car, and when I tried to stand up straight, the pain would travel in my spinal cord like one of those one hundred-mild-per-hour trains. The pain took no time to get to my neck, and then my neck and back would hurt quite a bit. I would walk around for a time to allow my back to loosen up, and then I would head into the house to lie down for a while.

I knew that it was time to get a good pillow to sit on. There were places I had to go to and where I must sit down. After I was done resting, I started looking for a good pillow for me to be able to sit on and hopefully cut the pain. This would become a huge factor for me, as I had to cut the pain sitting down as much as I could in case the time came when I was unable to sit. It would be a while before this was determined.

The next month I would be spending time at physical therapy and seeing all of my doctors again. I hadn't seen my psychologist or my psychiatrist in more than a month. The same was true of my pain doctor, and I had to get back to him so he could keep me going. I started back to therapy on each Monday, Wednesday, and Friday to see if I could build myself up again. I had been sloughing it for a while, and now maybe I would be on the road to success again. I was finally able to drive again, so I could make it to therapy without having to walk.

Among all of my appointments, I had to see my lawyers, as the lawsuit would be going to trial in the next few months. This was something I had to take care of, because just in case my life would not be the way it was, I need some security for the errors that had been created. This was not a problem of mine. I would be glad when this whole thing was over, as it was really bothering me mentally, and I worried about it quite a bit. If we could get this lawsuit taken care of, I would feel a lot better.

CHAPTER 24

My back was bothering me quite a bit, along with me neck. I was hoping that things would get better instead of worse. I noticed something new that day. I had begun to think about death, death again .

I did learn one very important thing. I went into the bathroom earlier in the day, and it was very painful. Also, I could not tell when I had gone in the toilet. I did not have any feeling of relief as I normally had had over the years. Something had changed in my back. I didn't know what it was, but I knew I had to find out what it was.

Over the next few days, I had the same thing happen twice more. I also discovered that I had to push on my stomach to be able to go, and that was beginning to change the way I lived. The doctor had told me at the last visit that I was probably going to have to live with the problems I was having. As time went on, other things were becoming more evident. I know now that this was the result of the back surgery, which I had no idea would happen. Another crazy thing that also changed was my sneezing. I no longer sneezed on a regular basis. I had kept track for a stretch of time and realized that I hadn't sneezed in three months. I felt this was very different. Other small things began to occur as well, but I just had to live with them.

I had to get my new bone growth stimulator, which I had to wear most of the day. The device would help grow new bones in my back. They have all kinds of different products on the market today to help after the back operation I'd had.

The following day I'd had an appointment with my psychologist and physical therapy. I had therapy three times that week, and that would be the same each week until I was told otherwise.

I had to go to therapy at nine o'clock in the morning and then see Dr. L at two o'clock in the afternoon.

Connie and I went through the day watching TV and taking it easy. I had taken my walks, and the next day I would begin to have my appointments and have to take my two walks too. Fortunately, I could drive now.

I woke up at seven and had to get ready for my first walk. Then I would have breakfast and take a shower before my therapy session at a quarter to nine. I would have to stay on my toes to be on time.

When I went to therapy, Connie was still sleeping. I got through my therapy, and when I got home, Connie was just getting up. I knew that she wanted to go to my appointment with Dr. L that afternoon, so she had to hurry so we could be on time.

We got to the doctor's office on time and had a good meeting with Dr. L. We had a nice long talk about my current health situation. I told him that things were not as good as I had hoped. But what could I do? Nothing at all.

When we got home from Dr. L's office, I was pretty tired, and I still had to take my afternoon walk. I finished my walk and then went into the house and crashed. This was the most activity I'd had since after my surgery

Many things had begun to happen to me, both physically and mentally, about a month after my back surgery. I developed a major problem with constipation where I would go into the bathroom and just sit down, hoping to go. Unfortunately, I always realized this was something that was not going to happen right away. Since I had little feeling in my back and never knew when I had to go, I would start by pushing my stomach in with my fingers. First gas in my stomach would exit at some point in time. I then would be ready to hopefully have a BM. Sometimes I went, and other times

I didn't. I tried to keep a daily record of what I would do, but it didn't work. It was a flip of the coin if I went or not.

There were times in the night when I've had to urinate. I would push on my stomach with no luck. Before I knew it, I had fallen asleep on the toilet. Two hours later, I'd get up and fall on my face due to my legs falling asleep. This has happened to me a couple of times since I'd had my surgery in January 2003. When I told Connie that, she couldn't believe it.

Other problems which I ran into were me straining too much to try and have a BM. I would sit there for many minutes, hoping that I could create a feeling in my stomach that I had to go to the bathroom. I was becoming very concerned about this, as I had no idea what I would do when I got older. Many things scare me about getting older. They are things I can only anticipate now, but it bothers me thinking about it.

I have also had a major problem finding shoes to wear. Everything I tried was very bad for my back. I went out and bought special shoes and tried sneakers along with very expensive driving shoes. All were no good for my back. I was in Walmart one day and saw these camouflage shoes that were very cheap. Just for the fun of it, I bought a pair, and I have been wearing them ever since. They felt so comfortable that I went back and bought two more pairs for when the first pair wore out. People would never think of what shoes can do to a bad back, and I sure found out.

The new air bed was great, but I found that my back pain changed depending on the type of day it was. For example, my back hurts worse when it rains, or if I really overdo it, I know I'll pay for it. I had to really learn how to use the air control properly. I was sure if I really learned how to use it, my back would feel better than it had.

CHAPTER 25

January 2004 was now upon me and my family. My neck and back had not gotten any better at all. I was dealing with a pain level of six to seven out of ten, depending on the day. If I had to ride into Rochester for my doctor's appointment, when I got out of the car, it could rise to a nine or a ten.

I knew that things would not improve unless I considered having another back surgery. After thinking about this for quite a bit of time, I decided not to go through with another surgery. It would be a fifty-fifty chance that it might work, and I was not going to take the chance again. My life was bad enough, and I wouldn't take any more chances.

I had learned to use my cane pretty well by this point in time. I couldn't believe that I needed this device to walk. I also had a grabber in each room of the house and outside in the garage. Using the grabber, I could pick things up off of the ground or floor without having to bend over. It has helped me so much, as trying to bend over had become very painful. I continued to go to therapy even though it didn't help anymore that I knew of. My surgeon and pain specialist wanted me to continue going, so I did.

I was still on the fentanyl patch, and there were things I couldn't do while wearing it. I couldn't go into a hot tub, and there were a few other things I couldn't do as well. The other thing that really bothered me was the possibility of becoming addicted to them. But I need them badly for pain. I also became very concerned when my pharmacy ran out of them for some reason. We then had to look all over for them. This scared me a couple of times, as there was nothing else I could take.

I finally came to the realization that I had to admit that I was in the class of a person with chronic pain. There was nothing else I could do other than surgery, and I wouldn't do that again. I again found myself thinking about dying, and why, I didn't know.

I knew that I had to keep going and try to do new things each day. If I was going to get back to the way I was before the accident, then I had to put forth an effort to build my body up again. I'd had this cane since my back surgery in 2003, and I knew I needed to really work hard so I could stop using this device, which made me look like I was one hundred years old. I know that I need it for the time being, but if I kept going on my rebuilding program, then I would be able to get rid of it once and for all.

I was really looking forward to returning to work, but at this point, I wasn't sure if that would ever happen. There were times I woke up in the morning after having a dream, and in the dream I never returned to work again. I really hoped that wouldn't happen to me. There were so many things I wanted to do both immediately and when I retired.

Each day of mine was the same as the day before. The only difference was the appointments I had for that day. The pain remained about the same. I had accepted the fact that I would never have a painless life again. Connie had done so much for me. Jen had been thinking about leaving Le Roy. After her second divorce, she decided to become a traveling nurse and travel across the country to Arizona. I knew that Jen and Connie had been talking about this quite a bit for several months.

The pain specialist from Buffalo whom I had been working with decided to go back to Buffalo on a full-time basis. Thankfully, a good friend of mine had a great pain specialist in Rochester, and we were able to go see him right away. This solved the problem of searching all over two counties to try and find a good pain specialist. Connie had made an appointment with Dr. N, and I would see him in three days.

Jen called us one night in late April and mentioned that she would be driving to Tucson, Arizona, on May 17, 2004, for her new job. Her moving date was just about three weeks away, and I knew she'd talked with Connie about this before. I knew that Connie would really like to go with her, but she was afraid to leave me by myself.

I had told Connie not to worry about me, but that didn't help her make this very hard decision. Jen was everything to us, and I really wanted Connie to make the trip with her. Jen's new job would start on May 24.

Connie finally made the decision to travel with Jen to Arizona, and I was very happy about it. I really hoped that she would go with Jen, and I knew that Jen would be very happy if she did.

I had several appointments before the time would come for Jen to leave. Most of the appointments were with doctors. I no longer went to therapy, as it had not been helping me at all. I had to see my new pain specialist doctor the week before Jen and Connie were to leave for Arizona. I also had four other doctors' appointments before they left. After that, I wouldn't have any appointments until Connie returned from Arizona.

My pain had been fairly consistent for a couple of weeks. I made it through my appointments, and it was now May 14, 2004. Finally, Connie committed to going with Jen. I was so glad that she would be going with her. Connie wouldn't have to worry about Jen driving by herself with her cat. We decided to have a pizza on Friday night to wish her good luck.

I knew that leaving would be hard on Jen, but she knew that she had to get away from everything happening around this place. She had gone through too much hell in the past few years. She'd had it and was getting out of here. Jen stayed with us for a while after her divorce and then with her very good friend in Bergen. I knew that I was going to miss Jen very much, as would Connie. She is such a great daughter, and all we could do was wish her good luck.

On Sunday, May 16, Jen was packing all of her stuff at her friend's home. She would pick Connie up at about ten o'clock the next morning for their trek to Arizona. It was going to be my job to man the computer and give them any information they might be looking for.

I really started to feel very bad that my baby was leaving Le Roy, and I wouldn't see her for quite some time. I also knew that Connie was very worried about me, and I had to do everything I could to make sure she wasn't concerned. I talked with the neighbors and asked them to tell Connie that they would watch over me while they were gone. They had told Connie that I would be okay, and they would look after me.

Connie finished her own packing and was ready to leave in the morning. We ate fairly late but had some very good chicken. I also bought macaroni salad, potato salad, and some French bread. We had a great meal, as I cooked the chicken on the grill, and Connie didn't really have to do anything but sit down. After eating, she went over things again to make sure she hadn't forgotten anything. Then she got dressed for bed, and I did the same. I fell asleep as soon as my head hit the pillow. I woke up at two and had to go to the bathroom. Connie had gone to bed, but I could see that her TV was still on. I went back to bed and woke up at six o'clock. I woke Connie up about a half an hour later.

The day had arrived when the ladies of the house were headed across country to Arizona for Jen's new job. Connie had showered and was ready when Jen pulled in about nine thirty. The car was packed to the roof. There wasn't an opening anywhere in her car for anything else after Connie's suitcases were put in. The cat had found little openings to be able to walk through the backseat like a tunnel. It was very funny.

I was talking with Jen for a few minutes when Connie walked out to the car. The neighbors from next door had walked over to wish them well on their trip. Both Connie and Jen gave me a hug and a kiss and then got into Jen's car. They said good-bye and then Jen started the car and drove down the street destined to the great state of Arizona. They were now gone, and I was alone.

CHAPTER 26

The pain I was living with sometimes seemed to have slowed down. I noticed that if my mind was on something else, I wouldn't think about how much I actually hurt. At times, I would see other people who I knew had a back or neck surgery, and I would ask them how they handled it each day. Much of the time the answer was that there was nothing else they could do but live through it.

At one point, I couldn't remember the last time I had really felt good. Connie and I used to go out with friends for dinner or just go to their house to talk and have a good time. We hadn't done that in about four years, and I honestly didn't know if we ever would again.

I belonged to the volunteer fire department, and each year there was a banquet we always went to. We hadn't attended since September 2000, and we really used to have a great time. But that was a thing of the past, and I didn't know if we would ever go again.

Unfortunately, Connie and I sat home every night with me in my bedroom and Connie in the living room. Now we never spent any time together, which hurt me, but what could I do? Connie didn't get out by herself much at all until this trip with Jen came up. I had hoped the trip would really allow her to have a good time, which she hadn't done in a couple of years. What an awful thing to say, but it was the truth. All she has done was take care of me.

I have struggled with problems in my life or even in our lives together, but I was facing something that I had no control of at all. I continually prayed and thought about things that I may be able to do to help the situation, but I had no answers at all. I had tried to read about things similar to what I was going through. I also sought out people who had lived like this before me.

No matter what I do, I begin to feel that my life is just about over. The things I had done over the years to give me enjoyment were now gone. As far as I knew, there was nothing else I could do or could go through that would give me part of my life back.

I decided that I should worry about Connie now. Her life had been thoroughly ruined, and I needed to find ways of getting her out of the house, such as this trip with Jen. But she would have to begin to enjoy her life again, and she couldn't worry about me any longer. She had done all she could for me. I was going to begin to think of things I could do to stop holding her back.

Connie was going to stay in Arizona for a week after they arrived. Jen would be with Connie for about four days until she had to start her new job. Connie helped Jen get situated, and then they drove around looking at the scenery. In the meantime, they also looked for rental properties in case we decided to spend the winter there. The time went by quickly, and before I knew it, Connie was ready to fly home. I talked with her the night before she was ready to leave, and I think that she would have liked to have stayed longer. My pain had really increased during the past few days, but I didn't tell Connie, as I didn't want her to worry. Something just didn't feel t feel right with my spinal cord stimulator SCS. Maybe it was all in my head.

I told her how much I loved her and that I missed her very much and then asked her how she liked Arizona. She told me that she really liked it and thought that I would also like spending the winter months there. She told me that she would see me in two days and that she really missed me. We said one last good-bye and hung up. Connie traveled by herself the next day with the realtor to look at a few rentals. Tomorrow, she'd be leaving for home. I talked with her and Jen briefly that night, and Connie was looking forward to coming home. I told them I loved them both and hung up.

Connie would be leaving Arizona today and arriving at the Rochester airport late tonight. Our friend Don would be taking me to Rochester to pick her up. We left at nine o'clock, as Connie's plane would be landing at around ten. Connie's plane landed at five after ten, and we met her at the gate. She looked so tired. We met her, and I gave her a big kiss. We then went to baggage claim and then to the car.

Finally, we were on our way home. I was really glad Connie was home again, but I was still worried about my baby. We drove for what seemed like two hours before we got home. I was just so happy Connie was home and wanted her in my arms, pain and all. Don finally pulled into the driveway and then helped bring in the suitcases before leaving. He said that he would call the next day.

Connie and I sat up for a while, and then Connie had to hit the sack. We had decided to talk in the morning. Connie went into her bathroom to do all her girly things. It would normally take her about a half an hour before she hit the sheets. All I did was lie on the bed , and within five minutes, I was out like a light. Of course, it always helped to take a Vicodin before going to bed.

I woke up at about eight o'clock and felt a toothache, which I hadn't had in quite some time. I hadn't had good luck with my teeth, as I'd had to have a few pulled in the last ten years or so. I brushed regularly but still had really bad luck. Then I thought about the dentist's chair that I couldn't sit in. It was very painful to my back. Between that chair and a flat table in the hospital for x-rays, I absolutely had so much pain when I was either in the chair or lying on the table. I decided to wait and see how the tooth felt a little later.

Connie slept until about eleven thirty, and she was very tired from the big trip, which had taken all day. I thought about the trip she had on the plane, and it really scared me if we ever went to Arizona. Sitting that long would kill me. But I wouldn't worry about it until the time came—if it came. When Connie walked into the living room, I could see that she was physically beat. Now she was home and could relax. I was very glad she was home, as I missed her very much.

I had her coffee made, and she poured a cup and then loaded it up with a little sugar and milk before taking a sip. She closed her eyes as she sipped her Folgers coffee, which she liked very much. She then walked into the living room with me and sat on the love seat. She began to tell me what a great time she'd had. We talked for about an hour. She was all ready to go to Arizona during the winter months if we could afford it. That would be a discussion for a later time.

I had thought about a possible trip to Arizona for the winter months and wondered if I would be able to make it by plane. I really didn't know what to think, but I also became afraid just thinking about it. I didn't know what to do or who to talk to about it beside Connie. That was where the pressure came in, and I knew that I was really going to have to consider it soon. What would I do?

Connie and I sat down, and she told me about the great time she had. Then to end our conversation, she told me she'd talked with a realtor about renting property for this coming winter. The news was a big shock to my brain. A surge of excitement pounded in my head. I really hadn't realized that I'd be facing this so soon. It was only about five months away, and I still didn't know what to do. I really was going to have to give this some thought.

We watched TV for the rest of the night. Jen had called to make sure that Connie made it home okay. They talked on the phone for about an hour and a half. Of course, Connie had to call her back so the expense would not be charged to Jen. When Connie hung up the phone, a small tear slid down her cheek. I knew she had just really realized that Jen was gone, and she wouldn't see her that much. I consoled her and also began to cry a little. I had to really consider making the trip to Arizona. I owed it to my wife for all of the help she had given me. Without Connie, I would not be here today.

I had gone to bed at about eleven thirty. I was pretty tired, but I was able to deal with the pain, although I didn't know why. Maybe it was because Connie was home, and maybe it was because I was thinking about going to Arizona, but something seemed to be helping me through the days with my pain. In any event, I thanked God for all he had done for me.

I woke up the next morning with the thought of flying to Arizona. I planned to make a call to Dan to see what our status looked like regarding being able to afford to make a trip to Arizona and rent for a winter. I honestly don't know if we could afford it, but for Connie's sake, I hoped we could. Dan called me back and said that we were good to go. I had given him all the preliminary figures, and he was happy with them. Dan was a great guy, and we really appreciated him. Everyone should have a financial advisor to protect his interests. I found out that you don't need a lot of money to have an advisor. I should have had one years before I did.

Needless to say, I was thrilled to discover we could afford to go to Arizona over the winter. My back was still bothering me quite a bit, though, and I was afraid of what the outcome may be. I was sure I would get over it.

It was that morning that I sneezed for the first time since my back surgery.

CHAPTER 27

Connie had made all of the arrangements with the realtor in Arizona to rent a home. She also made the plane reservations, and I found someone to look after the house. Our friend Don would take us to the airport and drop us off. Everything was set, and in two days, we would be in Arizona, although I was still worried about the pain I would have to endure getting there.

The day was November 8, 2004, and we would see Jen very soon. Connie and I had both really missed her.

We were almost finished packing and had to be at the airport the next morning at ten o'clock. We went to bed early, and I couldn't sleep all night long because I was too busy worrying. I knew the pain I'd been having. I knew that I couldn't sit for long. This trip would last about seven hours, and I feared the pain would be just awful. But this was for the family—and me too, as wouldn't kid myself at all.

At five o'clock in the morning of October 28, 2004 I crawled off of the bed . I was quite tired and hoped that maybe I would fall asleep on the plane. It was going to be nonstop to Phoenix, and then we had to drive to Green Valley, Arizona, which was about three hours south of Phoenix.

Jen planned to pick us up with a friend whom she'd met since she had been in Arizona. Connie walked into the living room at five fifteen, and I had her coffee ready. A couple of hours later, we were en route to the Rochester International Airport. I still had a funny feeling inside my stomach.

Connie had to get a wheelchair for me after we got out of the car. We loaded all of our baggage on the wheelchair. She was going to try to push me, but I found a skycap who was able to push me to the line for our airline. He got me through the line and then wheeled me to the gate where we had to board the plane.

The wheelchairs always entered the plane first, and there were three other wheelchairs ready to be boarded. After about forty-five minutes, we checked in and were able to board the airplane. I found a seat and then sat down. I was thinking about the pain I would have to deal with before landing. Fortunately, Connie had a pill to quiet me down. I took it, and about ten minutes later, I went to sleep. I slept most of the way to Phoenix with few problems.

Getting up from my seat was very painful. My back hurt very much, and the tears flowed down my cheeks. A man was at the plane's door with a wheelchair to wheel me up the ramp and to the gate. Our daughter was there to meet us in the waiting area.

We spent six months in Arizona, and the pain was off and on. The weather definitely made a difference. We spent quite a bit of time with Jen and loved every minute of it. The question was, would we go back again the following year? At that time, I didn't know. I pretty much stayed around the rental and didn't go many places unless I felt exceptional to do so. The stay was nice, and it did go by very quickly. We left Arizona on April 26, 2004, for New York, and I was really looking forward to getting back home and seeing everyone.

We arrived back in New York and began to try and plan our next few years. With the pain I continually lived with, I wasn't sure if we would ever leave Le Roy again. Depression began to filter into my life, as there was very little I was able to do around the house any longer. I had to hire out everything to be done. I didn't feel that I was worth anything any longer.

While we were in Arizona, we saw Jen about once a month and sometimes twice. Connie would spend at least one day a month with her shopping and having lunch together. Jen really loved it there. The months went very quickly, and before I knew it, April had arrived, and we were ready to fly back to New York and to our home in Le Roy.

The trip was very rough on my back. Connie had given me an ativan to help me get through all of the pain I had to deal with. After traveling about seven hours on the plane with two stopovers, when we hit Rochester, New York, I was crippled. The pain was unbelievable, and I couldn't wait to get home and lie on my bed. When we got home, I went into the bedroom to lie down. About four or five hours later, I felt much better. I didn't know if I could go through the experience again. I would have to really think about it for the next time.

CHAPTER 28

Connie had made an appointment with my neurosurgeon to talk about what else might be done. He suggested another surgery, but I didn't want to ever go through that again. I always remembered my good friend Jack telling me that he had nine back surgeries. I was all done with operations. I didn't know what I would do other than suffer as I had been since my back surgery in 2003.

I had gone through everything that was available to me. I had used all of the devices used with bad backs—every different vest or back support available, and nothing worked. Not even the surgeries worked after about two months. The pain was just eating away at my brain, and I didn't know what to do anymore. My life might as well stop, as I had no more ideas about what could be done.

Connie was also beginning to wonder what the outcome of my existence might be. We were fighting more and more, and it had come to the point that neither one of us had any positive feelings of me getting better. I had an appointment to see my pain specialist in two days, but I wasn't even sure I wanted to go. No one could help me any longer, so why waste my time and gas? The time went quickly, and Connie and I were on our way to Rochester to see Dr. N. We went into the waiting room and signed in. About five minutes later, we were on our way to one of the rooms.

When he came in, I broke down, as I was sure that there was nothing else for me to be rid of this rotten pain. He began telling me about a device called a spinal cord stimulator. This was the last chance for help. After explaining what the device does for the pain, he told me to think about it. I was as depressed as Connie was, and we no longer knew what to do. When we left Dr. N's office, we talked about it a little and then put it in the back of our minds. I seemed like just another thing that might make me feel a little better but only for a short time. I was not about to do that anymore.

The next couple of years were the same every week—going to appointments with my doctors, starting physical therapy back up, and doing everything that was told to me. But I didn't believe anyone any longer. Connie and I had a small relationship compared to before I fell and got hurt. All we did was argue with each other. My faith in God was almost nil. I never believed that I would ever feel any better and would just have to lie around the house doing nothing.

There was nothing worth living for any longer. My days would consist of me getting up at seven and walking around different Walmart stores in Batavia. I would then ride around for a little while and end up at Ace Hardware to get some coffee. I would then go home and do nothing the rest of the day. I would go into my bedroom, and Connie would spend her time in the living room, and that would be our day. Most of the time I would nap in the afternoon, and a normal meal at dinnertime never happened any longer.

Since my sister Rozella had passed on, my mother was splitting her time between her home in Florida during the winter months and my sister Sharon's home in Connecticut during the summer. She had an aid who spent twenty-four hours a day with her. I talked to Mom on the phone but didn't really see her that much anymore. I really loved my mom, but the pain I lived with kept me from doing many things.

I just felt awful every minute of every day. I had no life at all anymore. I would talk to my mom on the phone when I felt like it. I tried to call her every day, as she was still the strength that I needed to survive. Connie was my wife, and she had helped me so much, but my mother was the blood in my body.

I couldn't help but think, *God, my life is not worth living anymore with all the pain I have.* Maybe it was time I really thought about taking my life and not having to deal with everything any more. I couldn't handle anything. Connie had pretty much taken over everything. I used to pay all the bills and take care of the outside of the house. This was all a thing of the past. I couldn't do anything anymore, and I didn't care what the house looked like. Connie would do what she could outside, and then we either hired someone or my friend Don would come over to help. He would come over a lot to help—what a great friend.

I was not at all happy with the way my back and neck hurt. I was very concerned that the surgeries did not work the way that we had hoped. I was not about to go through any more surgeries, as I was already really skeptical about having the first ones, but I needed to do something to cut this awful pain I had. I was willing to do anything I could to cut or stop the pain, but I would never go ahead with another surgery again. I had realized that surgery doesn't always work. Although it worked with my first back surgery, I hadn't been as lucky with my most recent operations.

My life would never get better, and I had come to the point where I truly realized that. However, I would continue to search out anything I could to give me a cut in the pain I lived with. If I truly thought that I would never get better, then I might as well search out the best way to do myself in. I knew that I could not continue to live like this for the rest of my life. I would search everything I could to try and get better, but I was afraid that things seemed very hopeless at the time.

I wished that there were sites on the computer where I could go to get information from other people who had gone through the same things I have. It would help me so much, but I hadn't been able to find any. Chronic pain is a very critical situation that many people have faced or are facing now. I was told that I had a failed back surgery, and I know that I will never have another back surgery again. The pain is excruciating at times, and I am suffering so badly. The surgery was over a year ago on August 27, 2003.

CHAPTER 29

One morning I woke up and remembered some very weird dreams I'd had the night before. It seemed so real. The dream was about my dad, who had been gone since 1985. It was if he were right there with me telling me things I should do about my fall. He was not happy I'd been hurt, and he was going to go to my place of business and raise hell. It was if he knew what the outcome was going to be and wanted them to know that he was not happy with their commitment to me.

Many other things also came up in the dream. Although I can't remember everything now, I think when I woke up and realized it was only a dream, I wanted to cry. I miss him so much. There was so much more we could have done with each other.

My memory about the accident was very unclear at times regarding what happened and why. There was no need to do that work during regular hours. I should have let Connie sue the hell out of them. I had never asked for anything that wasn't due me. When I got hurt, it was like I had the plague. Few got in touch with me, and the only people who cared were the ones I had a good working relationship with. The major owner lost a son whom he was very close to, as were his wife and family. I, in essence, had lost my life with all of the pain and depression I have gone through. My marriage had not been good for the past few years, and I could not see where it would ever be back to where it was before I got hurt. I could not get out of my head being disabled all of my life. What had I done to create such ill feelings with someone? I had always been nice to most of the people I had ever met.

It was at this point when I began to seriously think about writing a book about all of my experiences. I wasn't sure if anyone would ever want to read it, but I knew it would be filled with a lot of things pertaining to living with pain every minute of every day. There were so many things I felt that I could share to help other people like myself. Why should they have to go through some of the things I went through when there is sometimes a much easier way?

I'd been to see so many doctors and specialists who felt they could help me. What a bunch of bull crap. No one could help me, and if they ever did, there would be the biggest party I'd ever had!

People often have no concept at all of what pain can do to a person unless they have lived with pain themselves for a long time. There are so many things that go through the head of a person who lives with continuous pain. In the beginning, you really don't care who understands. After a while, you pray that your family understands, but unfortunately, they don't. They don't realize that you can feel a little better one minute and the next you just can't handle it. This, to me, is one of the hardest things to try and get loved ones to understand. Reflecting back on the letter that was sent to me, I felt that after reading it, things would be okay, but it didn't turn out that way."

I swore to myself that if I ever got through this intense pain, which I don't think will ever happen, I would do my best to try and let people know what real pain is. The letter that was created a few years ago, was the best informative thing I had ever seen. Unfortunately, I found that people still do not understand if they haven't gone through it. I vowed to try my best to change that. I would also like to help people with some of the problems they may have.

I could see that my life would be limited as to what I could do. There are so many things I will have lost from this rotten accident. I am very fortunate, though. I could have ended up a paraplegic in a wheelchair. That really would have put me over the top. I just have to keep reminding myself how lucky I am. But how can you be lucky to live in deep pain every minute of every day? I have seen so many people in the same situation I am in, and the only difference in most cases is that my wife was a nurse. Connie had been such an inspiration to me.

Before I was operated on, I had more appointments than I could handle. Once I had gone as far as I could, there was nothing else to do and nowhere else to go. The only thing I wondered about in the back of my mind was laser surgery, and I was quite sure I would never go ahead with the procedure. It is somewhat like the regular surgery as far as taking a chance. I figured that I could go to therapy and any other thing that came along, and maybe, someday, I might find something to cure me.

Each day I got up I started to pray to God for his help, as I was to the point where I felt I might do something to myself. Connie and I had lost the true love we once had. Jenny had problems with her last marriage, which landed her in Arizona. This was another thing that had eaten at Connie. Her baby was no longer close to her, and she loved Jenny so very much. I felt that Jenny was the one keeping Connie and I together. With all the crap Connie had to face alone, she could turn to Jenny for support, but Jenny wasn't around anymore. Fortunately, Connie could talk to Jenny on the phone; they could talk for hours if they didn't have things to do.

When the summer began, I knew my sister and mother would be flying home to see me and the rest of the family soon. They tried to come home each year around our Oatka Festival Parade. During that time, there is a big parade, and craft shops are set up on the high school lawn to sell their goods. It is a great time in Le Roy once a year. Sharon and Mom would be home in a couple of weeks, and I was really excited. I didn't feel worth a shit, but seeing them would make me feel better mentally at least.

I was also able to talk to Connie about seeing a psychologist to try and get things off her chest. I hoped that she could get some help of her own. She needed it badly. She had been going to see my doctor, who was Dr. L in Batavia. We had both seen him a couple of weeks earlier. Connie was going to see the doctor in the next couple of days, and I had to go to my psychiatrist that following day.

I woke up the morning of November 20, 2004 with some chest pains. I didn't want to say anything to Connie until I was sure they wouldn't go away. I had an appointment in Batavia at two o'clock that I didn't want to miss. I waited for about an hour and a half, and when the pain continued, I told Connie. She immediately took my blood pressure and then called the doctor in Rochester. My doctor told her to have me brought into the hospital by ambulance. When Connie got off of the phone, she told me I had to go to the hospital and then she called the ambulance. About fifteen minutes later, the ambulance crew showed up and took my vitals and then loaded me into the rig. We were soon on our way to Strong Memorial Hospital in Rochester.

Connie followed in the car and got there about an hour and a half later. I was taken into x-ray immediately when we arrived. After the x-rays, I was taken back to the emergency room. I was given more tests there, and Connie eventually made it to the hospital and came into the emergency room. The doctor came in about an hour after Connie arrived and told us everything was okay. I was able to return home. I had not had any more chest pains after I got to the hospital, and I figured it was just indigestion. I was really glad I didn't have any problems, as I have had enough. Connie went to pick the car up and drove it to the back of the emergency room where I was waiting in a wheelchair. I got into the car, and we were on our way to Le Roy. Connie had called before leaving for the hospital to my psychiatrist and cancelled my appointment.

When we got home, I went to bed to relax for a while. I soon fell asleep and woke up about three hours later. Connie also decided to lie down and was still sleeping when I got up. I kept really quiet so she could sleep longer. She finally woke up at about six o'clock that evening and was kind of cranky. I stayed away from her for a while, and soon she was okay. I had put her through so much. It had been very unfair that I had to fall down those stairs due to incompetence, and our lives ended up being ruined. God does things in funny ways, and I guess I was one picked out to handle this particular problem. Don't ask me why, as I have no idea why I was the one picked out.

CHAPTER 30

I don't think that Connie's and my lives will ever be back to the way they use to be. We used to have some good times, but things were very different. This is a girl whom I loved with all of my heart and would do anything for. Unfortunately, she had to bear the brunt of everything in our home. It has not been fair to her, but what else could I do? My life had been ruined, and I was ruining hers. I wondered what would happen in the next ten years from now on November 23, 2014. I could see nothing good coming out of all of this.

My pain was constant, and we didn't do anything anymore. I sure wished that all of this were a big dream, but it wasn't. At times, I tried to compare my life to someone else's, but I could never think of anyone who was in a similar situation. I had felt sorry for myself for a good, long time, and it didn't do me any good to feel that way. With the pain I had been living with, Connie and I had no life at all. We spent almost every minute of every day in the house. Connie didn't go out at all except for appointments.

There was a time when I thought Connie was going to start going to the Red Hat Society. It was very hard to get her out, but I thought she was going to start going but never did.

I never went out much without Connie, like going to have drinks with the guys. I never liked going to bars or anything like that. I wished that I were able to take my wife somewhere, but with my back and neck, it was unheard of. I was not worth anything any longer.

I felt like my whole experience needed to be documented somehow, so what I had experienced might help other people going through almost the same thing. Between Connie and I, we had kept very good notes on everything I had been through and the feeling of pain I experienced. Over the years, I have my very bad days and then just plain old bad days and then sometimes good days. Normally, on my good days, I would try to do things around the house, then I'd overdo it, and then I'd suffer the next day. I have done a lot of praying along with the pain I have endured.

Our lives had changed drastically. Many of the things I used to do I could no longer do in many instances. Connie used to spend all of her time in the house when she wasn't working, and she now found herself concerned about taking care of me and making sure I was okay. We spent a lot our time together going to whatever appointments I had.

I was thrilled to have Mom and Sharon visit Connie and I for a few weeks. They were picked up from the airport at about nine o'clock and were staying at a motel. I couldn't wait to see them both—Mom especially, as her and I had always been very close. I told my dad before he passed away that I would always make sure Mom was taken care of. What a special lady she was.

When I knew they were settled in their motel, I gave them a call to say hello. I spoke to both of them, and they said they'd be stopping by the house at about three o'clock that afternoon. I really missed them and had even forgotten about this awful pain for a little while.

I told Connie that they were coming over, and we both got ready. It was ten o'clock that morning, and we had quite a bit of time to get ready before they came.

We were ready when they got there, and I held my mom for about five minutes before letting her go, as I did with my sister. We talked for a couple of hours until I had to go lie down. I went to the bedroom to lie down, and Connie sat and talked with them for another hour. Just before they left, they came into my bedroom to say good-bye. I couldn't believe that my mom had come to visit, and I had to lie down. Just because I can't sit or stand too long, I lost the chance to spend time with one of the most important people in my life.

Tell me that my life hadn't been totally ruined. There were so many things I had lost grips with, and who understood? Nobody did. No one had any idea what I had lost in my life because of stupidity of my company. Others sleep every night, but I don't. I couldn't help but wonder if maybe those people would read my book when it was done.

After Mom and Sharon left, Connie came in to see how I was doing. I told her I felt very bad, and I didn't know how I could handle everything much longer. I knew that my mom would not be around too much longer, and I had to come into the bedroom to lie down. I would never forget that as long as I lived. I didn't see how it could be any worse than this for me. Sharon and Mom were great to come and see us. Both of our families were fairly big, and the last time they came they stayed in Rozella's home but had since sold it. My mother meant so much to me. She had taken care of me my whole life, and I owed her everything. The problem was I couldn't take care of her any longer with the pain I was living with.

I would do anything for my family—anything. But unfortunately, while not feeling good, I was no good for anything. I was useless, and I knew it. This stupid accident, which should have never happened, had ruined my life and the lives of my family members. . How wrong I was to think that the major mistake I made by not letting Connie sue my company was the worst thing that could have ever happened to me. There was no way that I was going to be able to take care of all of these problems myself.

I should have gotten a lawyer in the beginning to get advice. If anyone ever asked me now, I would make sure and tell them that they need a lawyer. I have not handled this whole thing the best that I could. In the end, I have been totally screwed and lost a good portion of my life. The good things I had were gone forever. Connie and I were two different people. The love Connie and I once had for each other had now taken a new path. I had really not handled some of the problems we had correctly. I should have really gotten advice from someone, but with all the shit I had been dealing with these past few months, my head had not been straight. The drugs I had been taking for the pain really affected me quite a bit and hindered me trying to reason all of these things out.

CHAPTER 31

By November 20, 2006, I was so tired of living every day without feeling good. For whatever reason, I had been picked by my God to go through hell and to also put my wife, Connie, and the rest of my family through almost the same kind of hell. Every day I asked myself what I did to deserve this. However, I kept thinking about all of those poor servicemen who were fighting for our freedom every day. While they were being shot, stepping on land mines, and being killed in action, I was sitting back here whining like a baby.

Regardless what the pain is, millions have it every single day. In my case, I had to make some decisions. On top of everything else, the winter had been very bad, and Connie and I began talking about going back to Arizona to live full time. The cold was really creating big problems for me with the metal parts in my back aching an awful lot. This was another big decision that had to be made. I didn't know what to do, and I really needed God's help.

I had talked with my mom on the phone in Florida, and she was very concerned about me. She felt so bad that I was going through such intense pain. She didn't want me to have the surgery on my back in August of 2003, as she was very afraid. She thought I was very lucky with the surgery I had in 1986, which ended up working out fine, but she had bad vibes about this last one. She was definitely right, and I was suffering every minute of every day. I had no alternative at this point except maybe for the spinal cord stimulator, which I knew very little about. I was getting very lonely, and I wished I could see my mom. I think I could hold out a few more months.

My appointments with the doctors were less frequent near the end of 2006, as there was little that could be done with what I was living with. In my mind, I had only one chance left to help improve my life, and that was the new thing Dr. N had been telling us about. But I was really afraid and didn't know if I could go through with it. If it didn't work, I would have to spend the rest of my life in debilitating pain. Could I do it? I didn't know, and that is what scares me. There was no one who I could really talk with. I would have to do some more thinking and get serious about it.

The weather was becoming very cold in New York, and the steel in my back was really creating problems for me. There was no way I could feel better unless I hopped into the shower to warm the metal up. I was glad that I don't have an appointment with Dr. N that week, as the weather was supposed to be really bad, and Connie does not want to drive in the bad weather. I don't blame her.

I had an appointment with Dr. N the following week, and I was going to get serious with this stimulator device. There were many things I had to think about regarding continuing to live like this. Was it fair to Connie? If I could do anything to possibly improve my situation, I had to do it. I would continue to pray every night to get the answer of what to do.

Christmas was just a few weeks away, and I had no good feelings about the season. When you don't feel good, all you want to do is stay home and not see people. I hoped that Connie and I could get through this holiday all right, and then I could get back to my doctors and appointments. Connie and I talked about what to get Jen, and we both said we don't want anything. I was really tired on this particular day, and so I went to lie down on the bed for a while when the phone rang. It was Sharon. She had called to say that Mom had fallen and hit her head in Florida. Tomi, my mother's aid, had her taken to the hospital. I was really worried due to her age. I hoped that she would be okay, as I didn't know what I would do if she didn't make it through this.

Sharon called Elaine, and both planned to go to Florida as soon as they could. I wished I could go, and I even mentioned it to Sharon and Connie. They both told me to forget it. Sharon said that between her and Elaine, they would be able to take care of everything. I didn't know what to do.

Sharon and Elaine got there in two days and immediately went to the hospital. After they had spent some times with Tomi and the doctors, Sharon called me. She told me that Mom was not good, as she hit her head very hard. However, she also said that Mom could talk a little and asked me if I wanted to talk to her. I told Sharon I did, and she held the phone up to Mom's ear.

I said, "Hello, Mom. How are you doing?" Mom replied back to me in a very low voice that she didn't feel good. Tears began to slide down my cheeks, and at that moment, I became very concerned that she might not make it. We talked for a few more sentences, and then Mom had to stop. Sharon then picked the phone up to tell me that she was not good at all. In fact, the doctors didn't expect her to live more than a day or so.

I began to cry fairly hard and started to become very upset. *I must get to Florida to see Mom before she dies*, I thought to myself. *I have to see her.* Sharon told me to forget trying to get to Florida. She said that she and Elaine would take care of things. I told Sharon that I had to see her. She told me that mom wouldn't even recognize me by the time I got there; if she was even still alive. I told Sharon to call me back later if she would. I began to talk to Connie about going to Florida, and she told me that there was no way I could fly there. She also told me that they were having enough problems there without me going there and not feeling well. I agreed with Connie and decided to forget about even talking about it anymore.

A few hours went by, and the phone rang again. Connie picked it up. It was Sharon calling back. Connie and she talked for about fifteen to twenty minutes, and then Connie hung up. I asked Connie why she didn't let me talk to Sharon, and Connie explained that the doctor had just walked into the room and Sharon wanted to talk with him. Connie went on to tell me that Mom was drifting in and out of consciousness. I hated to even think such things, but I felt as though it was finally the end for my beautiful mother. She had meant so much to me over the years. She had given such love to all of us. I wished that Rozella were here with us, but she had to go before her mother. She loved mom so much also.

Rozella and I took care of Mom after Dad had died in June 1985. Before we took Dad into the hospital, he told me that he knew he would never be home again. He wanted me to make sure that I took care of Mom. I told him I would. Rozella and I watched over Mom for many years. Rozella would go over to the house each day to play cards with her. She would also take her to see friends of hers. Between Rozella and me, we had to tell Mom she couldn't drive any more. We also had Sharon and Elaine's help over the phone. Everyone loved my mother.

Sharon called back after the doctor left to tell us that Mom only had a few hours left. She had evidently fallen backward coming out of her bathroom and hit her head on a table. She had hit her head very hard, and her time was now here. Sharon began to cry, as did I. She asked me if I wanted to talk to her one more time before it was no longer possible. I told her I did, and Sharon put the phone up to Mom's ear.

Mom really had to force herself to get the words out, but she told me she loved me. I loved my mom so much. I prayed that God would take care of this great woman. Sharon then told me that she would call back a little later and keep me updated. Within a couple of hours, my mother, Rose Bean Scott, had passed away in Florida. The date of her death was December 21, 2006. What a great woman she was, and we loved her so much.

Shortly after Mom passed away, Sharon, Elaine, and I were talking about various things that had to be taken care of with regard to Mom's estate. Questions had come up on a few things, and one of the girls brought up the question of a will. Neither knew that years earlier in Le Roy Mom created a will with her attorney. Mom had made Rozella and me executers of her estate. I remember the reason was that both Rozella and I lived in Le Roy, and Elaine and Sharon lived far away. Of course, Mom never thought that if anything happened to Rozella, she would probably go to live with Sharon. In any event, I was the only remaining executor of her estate. Neither Sharon nor Elaine was ever aware that Mom had a will.

Things had come up regarding what was to be done with her personal items. My sisters had indicated to me that I should determine who in the family would receive these very loving mementos. Over the next week, Mom's body was sent home from Florida and was seen at the local funeral home. Her death absolutely created a living hell for me. The funeral home was only going to be open one day, and the people just flooded the place. She knew so many people, and there had to be more than two hundred people who came to pay their respects.

After everyone was done, the family went to say their last good-byes to such a wonderful woman. They broke the mold after making this most special lady. I wasn't able to see her in Florida to say good-bye, which really hurt me badly every day. I wanted to see her so badly but was unable to because of my back and neck. My mother was everything to me, and now she was gone.

She was finally put to rest on December 27, 2006. The love of our lives was now gone. I wanted to be in Florida with her before she passed, and I didn't go. I should have, and that will haunt me the rest of my life. I loved this remarkable lady so much. I should have been with her, but I wasn't. It is inexcusable that I wasn't there. It was my duty as her only son to be there before she passed on. I feel so bad inside, and I will never get over that.

Our Christmas with Mom passing was even less of a Christmas than we originally thought we would have. She was the pillar of our family over many years. Uncle Lloyd, who now lives in Hamburg, New York, idolized my mother. They were very close, and he took her death very hard.

Since Mom was now gone, Connie and I became more serious about moving to Arizona. The winter of 2006 had been awful and very cold. My rods and the other metal in my back and neck had created a lot of pain for me. Aside from this, Jen was still in Arizona by herself, and Connie really wanted to be closer to her. She had a rotten marriage, and it would be nicer if we could see her more than we did.

Connie and I had begun to sit down and put things on paper. Everything would have to depend on what happened with the spinal cord stimulator (SCS). This device is used to exert pulsed electrical signals to the spinal cord to control chronic pain. If I received the implant, and it worked, things would be a lot better. I hoped that things would turn out for us.

CHAPTER 32

A couple of months after my mom's funeral, I had finally decided to see Dr. N about the spinal cord stimulator (SCS). With the pain that I had been living with every minute of every day, I had to do something. I could no longer put up with it. Connie and I were also still considering a move to Arizona, and we needed to determine if it were possible. We didn't see the move as feasible without the successful implantation of the stimulator.

I asked Connie if she would call and make an appointment to see Dr. N, and she got something set up we could discuss the SCS in detail. My appointment was set the morning of February 28. Dr. N obviously felt I was a good candidate, as he was now ready to explain everything to us about this device. Despite the fact that the possible move to Arizona was on our minds, we didn't feel that we could say anything to Dr. N, as we didn't want to create any other possible problems now.

We just knew that we sure as hell couldn't move anywhere else unless I felt a lot better. There was simply no way I could fly on an airplane for seven hours in my current condition. The chronic pain had really done a number on me. A few years earlier when we flew back and forth from Le Roy to Arizona, I didn't feel half as bad as I did at this point. Our plans would entirely be based on this new device.

Connie and I didn't get out much during the next week. It was very cold and snowed every day. I didn't even go to Ace Hardware. It was just too cold for me. I didn't mind staying in the house, as I was warm and could lie down more. The only problem I had thought about was that I wasn't getting any exercise by walking around Ace. That had been my primary reason for going there each day.

I had been thinking a lot about Connie lately. I was so fortunate to have a family to go to if I needed to. She had no one at all. She had no one to call if she had a problem. I could call my sister if I had a problem, but Connie held everything inside, which bothered me very much. I often prayed, *God, please take care of my beautiful wife and help her deal with the problems that she handles herself.*

During the next couple of days, I stayed in the house and didn't go out at all. Connie had a couple of places she had to go; she needed to get out of the house and be with people whom she could talk to and laugh with. I tried to help by cleaning a little in the house, but unfortunately, just as soon as I got started, I had to quit because of the pain I had to deal with. When Connie came home, she did notice the couple of small things I had done and thanked me.

I had an appointment with Dr. N in a few days, and Connie tended to become really worried thinking about the weather conditions.

On the morning of our trip to Dr. N's office in Rochester, the weather was not good outside. I was sure Connie was really worried, but there was nothing I could do, because she wouldn't let me drive.

I had to think of all the things I was going to talk to the doctor about. I was really nervous thinking about this new device not working if I decide to go ahead with it. Connie decided to get into the shower, and I would follow her when she was done. It is really cold outside, about 10 degrees, and snowing. The roads should be okay, though, if we took our time.

When Connie was done in the shower, I got in. We decided to leave at about ten thirty. That would give us more than an hour to get to my appointment, because we really wanted to take it easy. After getting breakfast and finishing all we had to do, it was ten fifteen. I told Connie I would go out and warm the car up. I got into the car, started it, and made sure everything looked okay. The lights and gauges on the dash all checked out, and we were ready to leave. Connie came out, and we were down the road.

It took us about an hour to get to the doctor's office, and we were a little early. That was okay, though, as we didn't hurry at all. We decided to go in and use the restrooms before going into the office. After refreshing ourselves, we went into the office. I signed in, and Connie sat down while I paced outside the office. After about five minutes, Connie called me in, and we went into the waiting room. The doctor came in right away and asked how I was. I told him the same, but I had really been getting depressed. I told him I would like to talk about the stimulator he'd told us about before.

He began by telling us that it was on the same principle as the TENS unit I had used before. The TENS gave electrical impulses through the top of the skin to the area where the pain was. The spinal cord stimulator did the same basic thing but was directed at the nerve or nerves that were causing my pain. He went through all of the information on what it would do for me. He explained that I had to go through a trial for a week to see if the SCS would work well for me. He told us about the positives and the negatives and explained that he couldn't guarantee anything. He felt that at this point, I should give it a try to see if it helped me, because I had nothing to lose. We chatted for about another twenty minutes, and I told him I wanted to think about it a little more. He then gave me some information on it along with a disc to watch. I thanked him, and we left. We had made another appointment a month later.

Connie and I got in the car and talked about the SCS for a little bit on the way home. We both agreed that we had no other alternatives. We would talk about this a little more before any real decision would be made. About an hour later, we pulled into the driveway after a slippery ride home. I knew that Connie hated the drive, but there was nothing I could do.

By the time we arrived home, my back really hurt from the cold and the trip in the car. I got out and was all crippled up. I wanted to walk outside for a while, but it was too cold. Instead, I went right inside. Even though I was tired, I went to the computer.

I had decided that I was going to find out all I could about the SCS. The one thing I had forgotten was that Jerry Lewis, the comedian, had one implanted in his back. He was in very bad shape with his back for years before having the stimulator put in. He felt a lot better after having it done. I looked through every site I could find. My back was killing me, but I was going to go as long as I could. After reviewing many sites, I had to lie down.

I fell asleep for about three hours and ten had to get up for dinner. After dinner, I was back on the computer again looking at more sites for the stimulator. I wasn't going to stop until I was able to make a decision. I spent another two hours, and my back and neck were very painful. I finally asked myself if I wanted to live like this for the rest of my life. The answer was, *Hell no, I am going for the SCS.*

With my decision made, I began to make a list of all the questions I needed to ask the doctor. It was then I realized I hadn't even looked at the disc he'd given us. Maybe a lot of my answers are on the disc.

Connie had come into my bedroom just as I began to look at the disc for the SCS. We both sat there looking at this disc, and it was quite interesting. It really looked like I may have a good chance to feel much better if I had one implanted. At that point, I had nothing to lose other than the possibility that I might not feel any better after the implant. After that, there was nothing else to try or do.

Each day when I got up, I would go to the computer to see if any new things had been posted about the spinal cord stimulator (SCS). I did find that there were about two or three manufacturers of the SCS. Some devices had batteries that were good for five years, while others were different. I didn't know what manufacturer Dr. N had used in the past, and at that point, I didn't really care.

I was sure that my decision had been made. I was going to go through the trial test to see if the SCS would work for me. After talking with Connie, she agreed that I should try it. At that point in my life, Connie's input was a valuable part of my decision-making process, which is why I always asked her.

CHAPTER 33

On the morning of my follow-up appointment with Dr. N, I woke up early, as I was very excited to go talk about the new SCS. I was sold on it and was very nervous about whether it would give me the relief I had been seeking for so long.

I had prayed to God on a regular basis, telling him that if I felt good again, I would help him all I could with people who may need my help.

Connie and I got ready and took off at twelve thirty that afternoon. The weather outside was sunny and cold. The roads were bare, and I was sure that Connie felt good that it was going to be an easy drive to Rochester. After about forty-five minutes, we pulled into the parking lot. I then got out of the car and began to walk for about five minutes to help my sore back before heading into the office. My back and neck really hurt, and I was ready to finally take a chance on something new that I believed would help me. I was so excited about the move I was making to finally feel better. I stopped for a moment and wondered why I hadn't done this sooner. I will never know.

The nurse took us into the waiting room, and the doctor came in right after her. He asked how I was feeling. I told him lousy but added that I hoped that would soon change. I told him I was ready for the trial of the spinal cord stimulator (SCS), although I did have some questions for him, and I also wanted to know when we could do it.

He looked at his schedule and told me that he could do the trial on April 6, 2007, at eight o'clock in the morning. Connie also had a couple of questions she wanted to ask. The first thing she wanted to know was if we moved out of New York, would I be taken care of wherever we went. The doctor told us that I would be taken care of anyplace. I was very happy to hear this and couldn't wait to have it done.

I also asked which company he used for the SCS. He told me Advanced Neuromodulation Systems, which eventually changed its name to St. Jude Medical. My sister Sharon had decided that she wanted to be with us when the trial was done, so she could serve as moral support for both Connie and me. I really needed all of the support I could get, as I was very concerned about the outcome.

The next few weeks seemed to go by very slowly. It really wasn't dragging, but it felt that way. Connie and I had talked about this quite a bit, and it was all positive. I was really thinking about feeling better. I couldn't wait. Even though I had the pain in my back and neck, I knew that we were now on a time schedule for me to start feeling good again. I was so happy, and I thanked God every single day. He had done so much for me, and I owed him so much. But despite my excitement, the fear I had about it not working was really taking its toll on me.

I woke up one morning in a lot of pain. I began thinking about the last chance I had in life, for now, at least, to feel better. I realized that it was a coin flip, and it would either work or it wouldn't work. I had been in pain for so long, and I needed to take this last chance to hopefully give me a new life. I prayed every day asking God for his help in this matter. I told him that if this worked, my goal was to help any person who might need my help. If I could, I would be the person who talked about this device and tried to help others with a lot of pain. I would do all I could for anyone who felt that there was no help any longer.

I tried to keep a very positive attitude each day, but about five days before I was to have the trial done, I became very depressed. I started to think about things not working out as I had hoped. I had been having bad dreams that the trial did not work for me, and I was left at the end of the line. I feared that the pain would get even worse, and I would slide into a very deep depression and not care whether I lived or died. I was planning how to do away with myself without being caught, so Connie could collect on my life insurance policy. Unfortunately, the dreams I had repeated about three times, and I was really worried that they would come to be true.

Sharon was flying in to be with us and would stay at our house. She would be in town the night before the trial would take place, and I was so glad. Just knowing that she was coming helped get me out of my depressed feelings. However, the thought of her being there and the stimulator possibly not working was devastating to me. I wondered why I was becoming so negative when I had tried so hard to keep a positive attitude for so long. I knew the reason. It was a comment a good friend of mine had made about a year earlier.

He'd dealt with severe back pain much longer than I had. I talked with him about the stimulator and asked him why he didn't have the trial done on himself. His comment to me was that he couldn't bear it not working and knowing that was the end of the line for him. He would be in pain the rest of his life. Was he right? I wondered if perhaps I shouldn't go through with the trial.

Sharon flew in to the Rochester airport, and Connie and I went to pick her up. She was only going to be in town for two days. On the way home from the airport, we talked about the procedure that would be taking place. I began to get really nervous about the following morning. But the more Sharon talked about the SCS and what the outcome could be, the more I started to get very excited. I began with my positive attitude again, and it really felt good. I needed Sharon to tell me this.

Soon, we arrived home. Sharon would sleep in Jen's old room. As soon as we got in the door, I called and ordered a pizza to be delivered to us. It was great having Sharon with us, as I hadn't seen her in a few months. I knew her support would be a great addition to all that we had been through.

Sharon felt that being with us might help things turn out very positive and believed that I would end up feeling much better. I would take anything I could get at the moment. Could it be that God knew I needed her to be with me?

CHAPTER 34

Finally, the day of the trial had arrived. This would be the day of truth about the outcome and whether I would continue to have any kind of life. I had done all of the praying I could, and now it was in God's hands. I had cried and worried long enough. If I was going to suffer the rest of my life, I hoped I had the guts to do something to end it. I'd had enough and was very tired.

By seven o'clock that morning, I was up for the day. We had to be at the doctor's office by one o'clock that afternoon. Sharon was in the kitchen when I got up; she'd been out trying to take a walk in this very cold weather. She didn't go too far, though, as she told me she only made it to the end of the street and then came back. Sharon tried to walk any day that she could for exercise.

It was April 6, 2007, and I hoped it would be a day to remember.

I was very nervous and didn't know if I could make it through the procedure. I woke Connie up to make sure she would be ready. I had to go in several times, but she finally made it. It was now eight thirty, and we have to leave at by twelve thirty. I was starting to pray that this would work out. This was my last chance to hopefully reduce the pain. I had read many articles about the spinal cord stimulator (SCS), and there were a lot of good comments on what it had done for people. I just hoped that I would be another success story.

Should this turn out good for me, I would do anything to help other people. It has been so long that I couldn't remember what it was like to feel good. I thought that I had been a good individual through the years. I won't kid anyone, as I'd had my problems just like everyone else. But as a whole, I had been a good person. I couldn't help but think that one of the best things I could do to help people would be to possibly write a book on chronic pain. I wanted to try to explain to people what Connie and I had been through during the seven years since my accident. I knew that I had a lot to offer people if they wanted to read about this debilitating disease. It really can have an awful effect on a person, both physically and mentally.

Connie and I both got ready, and it was now about twelve thirty, and we were all in the car and on the way to the doctor's office. Having Sharon with us really helped me mentally. When we arrived, we were to go to a different building, which was where he performed the procedure for both the trial and permanent implants. Connie and I had not been in this building before, but we were about to get a good look at it.

As we pulled into the parking lot after a really cold drive, I got incredibly nervous thinking about the whole procedure. I think that Sharon could pick up that I was nervous and cracked a short joke, hoping to loosen me up. I kind of smirked at her and forgot the nervousness in my mind. We got out of the car, and my back really hurt. I had to walk around the parking lot for a few minutes to loosen my back up. The pain level was now about an eight, and I really hoped that this new trial worked to help me.

When we got into the office, I had to sign in. Soon a nurse came out to get me, and before I left, I gave Connie and Sharon each a kiss, and they both wished me luck. At that point, I was really worried. I was more scared than I had ever been in my life. If the trial worked, I would have relief, but if it didn't work, I would take the bridge. This is what it broke down to.

I walked behind this nurse, and she took me to a room where I could take my pants and shirt off. I then had to put on a gown that buttoned in the back. After I had my gown on, the nurse took me into a room that had about three or four beds. I lay down on the bed, and my doctor walked in

165

and explained what he was going to do. My blood pressure began to climb, and I had a very funny feeling in my stomach. He could see that I was very nervous and assured me that things would be fine. He told me he would see me in ten minutes. I thanked him as he walked into another room.

Then the anesthesiologist walked in and explained what he was going to do. He was going to give me a shot of medicine that would put me partly under. The reason for this was because the doctor needed to be able to ask me questions while implanting the wires. This helped him find the correct placement of the wires. He had to ask me when the stimulation reduced the amount of pain I was getting from the nerve that was causing the problem. As I was wheeled into the surgery room, I began to doze off. My worrying had ended finally, as I was now very tired.

Almost an hour later, I was ready to go home. I remembered the doctor asking me questions but I didn't remember what they were. The pain in my body had not changed as I had hoped. I was a candidate for the stimulator, but the implant did not work. I had waited so long to get part of my life back, and it didn't work. I couldn't help but wonder what Sharon and Connie would say when they heard the news. I began to cry and felt really depressed. What had I done in my life to suffer with all of this? My God, why was I still living? I could not handle this anymore, and I wanted to die—right then, I wanted to die.

Dr. N walked into the room and saw the tears rolling down my cheeks. He asked me why I was crying. I told him that I wanted it to work so much, but I continued to have the same pain. He then explained that the unit hadn't even been programmed yet or even turned on.

I couldn't believe my ears. *What did he mean it hasn't been programmed yet? Had I missed something that I don't remember someone telling me?* I thought to myself. I asked him to explain what he meant. He then told me that the sales representative from St. Jude Medical had to program my new unit with his programmer before it would work. I was so relieved. I thought I had missed something when he explained things to me, but I still had some of the drug inside me from the implant. I had thought that when I came out from the procedure, I would be good to go with regard to the new implant. But as the doctor explained, this was not true. *How could I be so stupid?* I wondered.

The doctor had me put into a wheelchair and taken to where the sales rep would program my new unit. Someone had gotten Connie and Sharon to meet us there, so they could see the programming as it happened. It would only take about fifteen minutes, but it was something they wanted to see.

As I was helped out of my wheelchair to a gurney-type cart, the sales rep took his unit out and grabbed hold of mine. He began to ask me questions as he was programming my unit. He wanted to know when the pain was reduced and if I felt better with the stimulation he had programmed in the unit. It took about fifteen minutes until he was done inputting about five programs, and then he wanted me to turn the unit off and then on again. As I did this, the feeling I had was unbelievable to describe. The horrendous pain I had lived with for so long was now better. It was another fifteen minutes after the programming was done that I was able to put my pants and shirt on.

The feeling that I had was indescribable to anyone that may ask at that given moment. I had to be the happiest man on the planet. My wife and sister looked at me, and by the expression on my face, they knew that everything was just great. They both wrapped their arms around me as they laughed and cried. After seven years of living with intense pain, I had something that finally gave me great relief.

At that moment, I looked up toward the sky and said, "Mom, I love you so much, and now I feel a lot better." My life was finally better.

For the test unit, I had several wires hanging beside me. But when the permanent unit was implanted, all the wires would be inside my body.

We had stayed at the building for about an hour after I had the programs set up. The doctor gave me time to really feel good about what I had just received—my new life. I would do so many things to now help other people. We finally left the building and headed back home. Everyone was happy but not as happy as I was. I had waited so long for something really good to happen to me, and it had finally happened. I did believe, and now it finally had happened.

Thank you, God. Thank you, God, was all I could think of. I felt him on my shoulder, and I knew that things would be better. As we traveled home, I had to call my baby in Arizona and give her the good news. We spoke for about five minutes, and she told me she loved me, and I began to cry a little. I told her I loved her so much, and then we hung up. I knew that Connie would give her a call when we got home.

As we pulled into the driveway at home, I still couldn't believe what had just happened to me. I felt better, and I could not believe it. I felt like when I was a kid at Christmas, and I couldn't wait to get downstairs to open gifts. This was the best gift I could ever imagine. When it was time to go into the house, I remembered that I didn't have to walk outside the car before going into the house. I no longer had to loosen up after riding in the car. My back felt good. I still did feel pain, but with this strange sensation now inside my body, it wasn't a pain level of seven or eight. Instead, it felt like it was about a three. It was relief.

When I got inside, I went to the couch to lie down. Connie and Sharon were getting drinks in the kitchen. I just lay on the couch and thought about how fortunate I was. The pain wasn't gone, but I definitely felt better. I had Vicodin to take in case the pain became greater than it was at that moment. I knew that I still had to take the drugs I was on, as they would keep me feeling good. I mustn't change anything at this point.

I had to go back to the doctor in a week to get the permanent implant done. If I had any problems, I was to call before that. At that moment, I was ready for the real implant. Jen had called back on the house phone and asked how I felt, and I told her great. She was so happy for me and was hoping that this would make it much easier on me if we moved to Arizona. Jen and I talked for about five or ten minutes, and then Connie and Sharon talked with her for a while. I could tell that Jen felt very good about what had happened to me. It had been so long.

Sharon came into the living room and gave me a big kiss. She also was very happy for me. She had helped me so much by just letting me talk to her when I was down. She was always so cheerful and positive about what was going to happen to me. Sharon had helped the whole family more than anyone would ever know. She took care of Mom after Rozella passed away and I got hurt. She took care of everything. She had her own family, but she still jumped in and took care of business—what a lady, first class all the way.

Sharon would be leaving at four o'clock the following afternoon, so we had to have her at the airport by two. When she got home, she would be there a couple of days and was then flying to California to see her son Tim and a couple of his kids. Her kids were the best.

A few years earlier, when I had just gotten out of high school, I decided to work at Strong Hospital in Rochester. Sharon and her husband, Wayne, lived in Rochester. They offered up their home in Rochester and let me live with them while I worked at the hospital. This was how I became so close to her family. The kids were just like my kids, and I loved them all as if they were my own.

Since they had moved to Connecticut, I hadn't seen that much of them. But as time went on and the kids got married, we traveled to Connecticut to attend the weddings. We were definitely very close to the Collins family.

After we all rested for a while, Connie got dinner ready. I would still have my food in my bedroom, as I had for several years. Sharon and Connie would sit in the den and talk for quite some time while eating. After dinner, they did the dishes and then sat down to relax. It was about seven o'clock, and I was going to watch few programs on TV. Sharon had to make some phone calls, and Connie sat down to read her book.

Sharon and Connie stayed up talking for a time and went to bed around midnight. I felt good going to bed for the first time in more than seven years. I still had to take a Vicodin before going to bed, but the pain was not as bad as it has been in the past. I knew I would still have to get used to changing the programs on the unit depending how I felt during the day or night. I prayed to God before I went to sleep and thanked him for all of his help.

I still couldn't believe that I felt as good as I did. I had to put things in perspective for people I talked with. It was similar to having a toothache along with a big gas pain. The toothache had gone away, but I still had the gas pain. The pain had basically been cut in half, and that made a very big difference with me.

I fell asleep and got up during the night to go to the bathroom. I then went back to bed. I woke up at about seven o'clock still feeling pretty good. My pain had increased somewhat, so I had to again read about using a different program that the sales representative had set up for me. When I read the instructions, I changed the program and again felt as good as I did when we left the doctor's office the day before. After reprogramming, I went to the kitchen where I found a note from Sharon saying she was out taking a short walk.

When Sharon returned from her walk, I went in to wake Connie up. Sharon and I then began to talk about what had happened to me. She still could not believe that I felt as good as I did after the trial was complete. She saw me go in with pain written all over my face and come out when it was done laughing. This device was something else, and I still could not believe it.

My situation with the stimulator was that I still needed the fentanyl patch to take care part of the pain that the stimulator didn't help. I also had the Vicodin to take care of any additional pain. I started applying the fentanyl patch every third day. As the pain began to get worse, the schedules changed. Finally, I was able to maintain my comfort level by changing the patch every other day.

The stimulator wires and the stimulation inside my body were going to change my life drastically. I needed this new life, and I hoped that it would continue. This new outlook changed many things I had thought of over the past couple of years. I had begun thinking more and more about suicide, which really scared me. The more I thought of it, the more scared

I became. Fortunately, I had been given ativan quite a while ago, and I took them as needed to get through this damn depression. I knew that I had to get that thought out of my mind. With this great breakthrough, I knew that things would change. I had to keep a positive attitude, and felt that moving forward, I was really going to feel good.

I began feeling very tired and decided to skip dinner. All I wanted to do was lie down. Again, Connie and Sharon began talking, and I thought that it was a good thing. Connie really didn't have anyone to talk to other than Jen and Sharon. After lying down, I finally woke up at about two o'clock in the morning. I couldn't believe that I'd slept so long. Sharon and Connie had gone to bed. Sharon was going home, and I wouldn't see her for a while. She had been extremely uplifting for me.

Sharon was up early, and I had just gotten up at about five o'clock. I walked into the kitchen, and there she was. I greeted her and then walked over to her, grabbed her, and hugged her. I told her how much I cared about her and how happy I was that she made time enough to come and be with Connie and me while I had the stimulator put in. Sharon had always been this way. She was always concerned about her family.

Sharon sat down and I stood up as usual, and we talked about our family. How lucky we were to have come from such a lovable family. I just thanked her for all she has done for me. Sharon had always been there for me. She had done what she could for everyone, and she was a carbon copy of my sister Rozella. She cared about everybody, and I loved her so much for that. She was such a caring person. We had talked for about an hour before Connie came walking into the kitchen.

I was feeling great with the spinal cord stimulator (SCS). The stimulator had given me a relief from the intense pain that I have lived with since 2003 after my surgery on my back. When you live with continuous pain for a number of years, anything can change the way you feel in life. My whole life was being based on this new device giving me a new feeling in life, and I honestly thought that it was my new breakthrough.

Sharon and Connie sat down, and I went into my bedroom to reevaluate my feelings of this trial. I still could not believe that I had received such relief from the intense pain I'd had. I really understood how so many people who have lived with chronic pain felt when they discover a new way of living a better life. This was a story that I was going to have to tell if it continued to work like it has.

The morning went fairly slowly, but we knew we had to take Sharon to the airport and had to start getting ready. It was now eight o'clock, and I had already taken a shower, as had Sharon after she'd gotten up. We started to get some breakfast ready, while Connie was taking a shower. Sharon was excited to be going home to see her family. I told her that I could never repay her for all she had done for me. Then we both began to cry, as I had said, "Mom is so happy right now." We loved our mother so much, and it was hard ever holding anything back when we talked about her.

After our breakfast, Sharon went in to pack her things, and I went into my room to get ready. Everything was still working fine, and I knew that this SCS was a big find for me. I had found new life in this small unit that gave me electrical impulses. Connie had walked into the room after getting out of the shower. I had finished what I had to do, so I wanted to get out of her way. She went into the bathroom to finish getting ready.

It was fairly cold outside, and I decided to take the car out for a ride to warm it up. I told Connie and Sharon I was going downtown for a minute and would be back. I had to hide all the wires that were hanging outside my pants. I drove around for about twenty minutes and then returned home. When I got back, Connie was getting some breakfast, and it was ten o'clock.

Sharon had everything packed, and we decided to leave at about eleven. We sat down after Connie ate and chatted for a while before leaving. Sharon asked me how I felt, and I told her that I was doing okay. There was no way that this stimulator would take the place of my fentanyl patches or my Vicodin. It was meant to hopefully reduce the drugs I was taking. Some people had gotten off of the drugs, but in my case, there was no way that would happen.

A few minutes before eleven, I started loading Sharon's suitcases in the trunk of the car. The weather was not bad out, and the roads were clear, so Connie was not worried about the drive to Rochester. We got into the car and were off to Rochester. It was going to be another test for how my back felt after getting to Rochester.

It was about forty minutes later when we pulled into the airport. Connie had pulled into short-term parking, but Sharon wanted her to drop her off in front. We wanted to walk her in. After she parked, we got the suitcases out of the trunk and went into the airport. We got to the desk so Sharon could sign in and then went to the security gate. We kissed her good-bye and waited for her to get through the gate. We waved, and she was gone down the hallway.

Connie and I went back to the car and drove home. My back was fine when we got to the airport, and now we would have to see what it was like when we got home. When we pulled into the driveway, Connie parked the car in the garage. As I got out of the car again, I realized my back felt pretty good. I didn't have the intense pain I used to have.

We went into the house and relaxed. It was then that I decided to call my sister Elaine who lived in Colorado, and I would update her on all that had just happened to me. I had forgotten to call her before, and that seems to be the standard for me. Since Elaine left our area and moved to Colorado, she hadn't been home much. So seeing her as little as I did, we didn't keep in real close contact. I think we were both to blame for that. In fact, I'd never even met some of her children. It had been hard for me to get close to anyone but Elaine, her husband, and their oldest daughter, Lori Beth.

CHAPTER 35

My life had completely turned around, and I had a reason for living again. When you live with pain every minute of every day for so many years, the life you lead is not worth even talking about. The friends you once had and saw fairly regularly change, and you no longer see them much at all. It wasn't that they weren't concerned, but I just didn't care to see anyone anymore, and I didn't want them to come and think they had to stay for an hour. It was really better for me that they all stayed away. It was very hard for Connie, as she didn't see hardly anyone any longer. Her life had taken the same road mine had, which was to be alone.

I was preparing to have the permanent implant done is just a couple of days. Each thing I did was much better than before I had the trial stimulator. I still could not believe that I had something worth living for. Maybe someday I could be involved in some type of group with people who suffered with chronic pain.

If this stimulator was the real thing, I would gladly meet with people experiencing the same things I had been through. It sure seems that I told God that I would help any way I could with the people who live in pain daily, and I would. It was the least I could do for gaining this new life.

Each night when I went to bed, I left the SCS on. I would have to reduce the stimulation, though, as it was pretty powerful lying down. Standing up, however, it was just fine. I had several of my friends who stopped by the house to see how I was doing. I felt pretty good compared to before I had the stimulator. All the people were really happy for me and hoped that the final implant worked just as well.

My appointment for the real implant was in two days. I was not going to really be happy until the final implant was done. I would get very happy when the implant was done and worked great. I was getting excited that my life would really be good after the final implant was done.

Connie and I had been through so much together, and I owed her so much. We had been talking about moving to Arizona, and everything seemed to be falling into place. We knew there was still going to be a lot of work ahead of us. We would have to sell our home without a realtor, because we needed to save all the money we could. Connie would have to make a trip to Arizona to look for a home if we really decided to make the move. I didn't think that I would try the flight, and she would be able to spend time with Jen. We knew this was something we were really going to have to sit down and think about.

Before I realized it, it was the day before the appointment to have my permanent implant. I was getting a little excited. I couldn't wait to get it all over with. Connie and I had a small dinner, and I decided to go to bed early. I wanted to get a good night's sleep if I could. I got my pajamas on at nine thirty and gave Connie a kiss good night. She asked me how I felt, and I told her I felt pretty good. She asked me what my pain level was, and I told her about a five. I had done a few things that day I probably shouldn't have, but I enjoyed doing them. I felt okay and ready to get the final implant done. I asked her what time she wanted to get up. She told me about seven o'clock, and I told her I would wake her up.

I slept fairly well during the night. I had gotten up a couple of times, once to go to the bathroom and the other just because I was nervous and excited. I eventually went back to bed and got up in time to wake Connie up. I had her coffee made, and she was wondering what the weather was like outside. Fortunately, it was okay outside, and the sun was out. I told her everything was okay, and she gave a sigh of relief. She really didn't like the snowy roads, and I didn't blame her. The weather in our area could be really crappy. I wished I could take a shower, but I couldn't, so I just washed up. About an hour later, Connie had gotten into the shower, and we had to leave at about eleven thirty, as our appointment was at one o'clock.

The time went slowly, but I was ready to get in the car and leave. We still had an hour and a half, so I decided to go outside and take the car for a ride to warm it up. We had a full tank of gas, and everything was okay for our big trip to Rochester. I had driven around for about thirty minutes and then came back home and parked the car in the garage. The sun was very bright, which was a good sign. I went back into the house and watched TV for a while until it was ready to leave. Connie had asked me if I was going to get something to eat, and I told her no. My stomach was too jumpy to eat. I would be fine until after the implant. She decided just to let it go, as she knew how I felt inside—very excited and like a kid at Christmas.

It was nearly time to go, so I went out to warm the car up again. Connie had told me she would be right out, and five minutes later, she walked into the garage. She got in the car and put her sunglasses on, and we took off to Rochester. I had said a little prayer as we were driving down the road. I prayed that everything went well. After about fifty minutes on the road, we pulled into the same parking lot we had been at a week earlier. My excitement had increased, and I was also scared. I didn't know how I could have two different feelings inside at the same time, but I did. Soon, this would be the moment of truth for me. The new implant would be in my back, and I'd feel the relief from pain from now on hopefully. This, by far, was the biggest thing for me since I'd fallen down the stairs on October 3, 2000.

The day was May 9, 2007, and in about three hours I would walk out of this doctor's office with the SCS fully implanted in my back. I would be a new man with a brand-new life. When I got inside, everyone was there, and I was ready for the final implant. I had to get into my gown, and the IV was placed in my arm. I gave Connie a big kiss, and then Dr. N walked in and asked if I was ready. I told him I was. The nurse beside him gave me a shot for me to doze off into neverland.

As I was being wheeled to the room where the full implant would take place, I began to fade in and out. The doctor had again told me that he would be asking me questions as we continued on with the implant. He had to once again find the nerve that was giving me all of the problems. Nearly two hours had gone by, and the new implant was all done, including the programming for my new unit *Thank you, God.*

If my stimulation remained at about four or five on the pain scale, I felt my life would be all set. The sales rep has given me about six different programs to use with my programmer. I would use them as needed. They were all different and controlled the pain in my back and both legs in different ways. I did have the added bonus of the stimulation going up my spinal cord to my neck. This was great, as I had quite a bit of pain in my neck area also. I had never thought that I would ever have a chance to feel better.

My pain level in the past had been as high as ten-plus, which was unbelievable, but I lived it. I realized what a lucky man I was. My life had taken a huge step in being able to live again without always thinking about suicide.

To me, the SCS was a lifesaver, as the pain I had lived with for more than seven years had been just awful. But now I felt much better. The pain was not completely gone, but at least I could tolerate it, which I had trouble doing before. The new life I had would improve a lot of things. I was so happy, and my God did not let me down. He gave me the maximum amount of pain I could live with, and just before everything crumbled, he gave me new life. I honestly believe that this was all intentional so I would decide to write a book on what I had been through during my life with chronic pain.

CHAPTER 36

The spinal cord stimulator (SCS) had given me a life that I never thought I would have again. I knew I would learn to cherish the final outcome of my life so far. I have so much that I could tell people who think that their lives are finished. They have to remain positive and not give up. With the spinal cord stimulator (SCS) and the different pain pills I take, my life was great. I didn't know if I would ever get off of the extra pain medication, but I was willing to wait and see as my life continued on.

I couldn't thank Dr. N enough for all he had done for me, as well as the sales representatives for the stimulator. I wish I had a lot of money that I could give them. I was so happy, and I knew I'd never forget that moment in my life.

Connie and I had thanked everyone at the doctor's office and got ready to leave for home. I had some phone calls I had to make, and we had to start preparing for our move to Arizona.

I discovered that many things were better with the new device in my back. I had to carry a card in my wallet, because the device may set off the alarm at airport security checkpoints. If that happened, I would have to show my card. I also had to get my medic alert bracelet changed to show that I had a stimulator, as there are certain procedures, such as an MRI, that I can no longer undergo.

I was going to have to get use to a lot of new things. I had to make sure I didn't overdo things and hurt my back. I was sure there would be times when I would overdo it, but I would learn over time. The full impact of what had been done for Connie and me had still not fully sunken into my very hard head. I had new hope for my life, which I never expected.

I thought back about four or five years earlier when all I thought about was taking my own life. At that time, I'd never heard of a spinal cord stimulator (SCS) and thought for sure that my life was useless. If there was only one thing I could do through the upcoming years, it would be to let people know about this great device.

My God in heaven put me through all of this so I could help spread the word about this great medical device that gave me back part of my life. I was so happy, and my whole attitude had changed—I mean, really changed a lot. I felt like one of the proudest and happiest men in the world, and I planned on helping as much as I can to let people know about this most unbelievable product that is in the marketplace today.

I wished so much that the family I lost was here to see me and how I felt. I began crying thinking about all Connie and I had been through. Our lives were all screwed up for a few years, and we never, in our lives, ever thought that this would all end up okay. I must be someone very special, because the one thing I know for sure is that I will never let this go until many people are aware of this.

CHAPTER 37

When we arrived in the driveway, I moved from left to right, and my back still felt great. It hurt a little but nothing like it had before the implant. This thing was great, and I was ready to talk about leaving the place where we'd both grown up. We went inside the house, and Connie noticed that the answering service had picked up a message. She walked over to see who it was when the phone started to ring with a brand-new call. She picked the phone up and discovered it was our fantastic daughter on the other end of the line. Connie handed the phone to me, and Jen congratulated me on my new implant. I thanked her very much and told her we might be on our way to Arizona. She was very happy to hear our news. She told me she loved me, and I handed the phone to Connie so she could talk to Jen.

Yes, it was now time to get very serious about moving to Arizona. Connie was very enthused about leaving Le Roy and being closer to Jenny. We loved our family and friends in Le Roy, but we also loved our daughter very much. The weather would also be much better for both me and Connie. Aside from all that, Connie was really high on leaving Le Roy and being by our only child. I felt the same way. There were many things we had to talk about in the next few weeks and months in order to be able to make the move that same year. We didn't want to stay another winter in New York even though we'd just spent quite a bit of money in the upkeep of our house. We'd put in some new tile floors, and I bought a home generator not even a year earlier in case the power ever went out in the very cold months of the winter.

I really felt good each day I got up. I did overdo it on some days, and on the following days, I really hurt and paid for doing too much. There was going to be a lot of work that needed to be done to the house, which Connie and I would have to do ourselves. I was not going to ask for any help until we absolutely had to.

We soon found ourselves at the end of March, and we began to really get going on selling our house and getting prices of movers to transfer the household to Arizona. The first thing I had to do was contact a couple of realtors to determine the value of our house. We'd bought it in 1968 for about $16,000 and had made many improvements since then.

A couple of days went by, and one of the realtors was due to stop by the house to talk It shouldn't take long, as I had a lot to do. I was feeling pretty good and would have felt better had I not pushed myself a little more than I should have.

The doorbell rang at one o'clock with the first realtor stopping by. We chatted with the realtor, who also happened to be a friend of ours, for about an hour, and I thanked her for all of her help. This is why we have good friends. She helped me out as a friend, and I would help her any time I was able if she needed something. Before leaving, she asked me if she could get a couple of brown boxes, and I told her I would have them in a couple of days. When she left, I called another friend at my former place of employment and asked him for a couple of boxes with the dimensions I gave him. That same night he stopped by with the cartons I had requested. My realtor friend had them the next day. She was very happy and couldn't believe how quickly I was able to get them for her.

The second realtor called me on April 5, and we set up a date for him to come to the house to talk about the price and sale. He mentioned he would be at the house the next day at one o'clock. This was also done at the time agreed on, and I had all the information I needed to sell the house myself.

I was now excited, as I knew with my experience that we could sell the house ourselves and save quite a bit of money. I finally felt comfortable about putting our house on the market, although we still had to do a couple of things before listing it.

I felt good for the next few days. I had an appointment with Dr., L to sit down and discuss how I'd been feeling. We talked for about an hour, and he was very happy to hear the way things had finally turned out for me. He was kind of surprised that we were going to go through with selling our home and moving to Arizona. I had talked to him about it but was not sure at the time, as it was before the implant of my stimulator. He saw how well I felt with my new appliance in my back and wished us all the luck in the world. I didn't know if I would be back to see him before we left. It would depend if I felt like I needed to talk to him.

Connie and I had so much to do to prepare for a move. However, Connie deserved this and everything else I was able to give her. She had taken care of me for so long, and I would do anything I could for her. I owed her my life. It took some time to get the posters and papers taken care of regarding the house sale. If we did things right, I felt that we could sell our house within a couple of months. I had to take my time and be good at what I did, and we should have no problem.

We also had to coordinate a garage sale, which would be fairly big. I kept thinking, *Thank God for my stimulator, because this is the only thing that will get me through all of this.*

We have a lot of things to sell to the public. Next, I would have to coordinate with the moving company. I hoped I got everything right so we didn't have any problems. We didn't need any problems along with this. Connie and I had both worked very hard to put all of this together. I could not believe that we had done so much over the past couple of months.

My SCS had truly been a godsend, and I felt so lucky to have one. My God above looked down on me and said, "Here is a guy who has been through a hell of a lot of pain over the past six months. Let me give him strength to feel better for these few months so they can do what has to be done to get to Arizona to be near their daughter."

One of the final steps was to create an ad to be put into the local paper in Batavia and also in the Le Roy *Penny Saver*. We made a great ad and finally got things going.

A good friend of mine, Dave, was able to get chairs and tents for us to use in our garage sale. Things really went well. It was very hard on both of us, but we got through it. Connie and I were really so tired from all of this, and at times, my back really hurt. Unfortunately, at times, I was doing things I never should have done, but there was no one else around to help me when these things had to be done. We continued to work our asses off until it was all over with. The garage sale was much bigger than I ever thought it would be.

My back would bother me quite a bit after the day was over, as I had pushed it way too much. I was warned about doing that, but things had to be done. With the garage sale all done, I had to slow down. I had some guys coming over to get all the material out of the garage that I was unable to reach. It didn't take long, and they got it all down.

It wasn't long before we had a couple from Batavia who were very interested in our home. They had looked at it once and were coming back again the following day for one more look. Connie and I were very excited that maybe we would have our home sold. The night went very slowly, and we talked for a long time about leaving this beautiful community that we'd both been raised in. It was now about eleven o'clock, and I was very tired and decided to go to bed. The next day would finally tell the story if our home would be sold.

I woke up at about five o'clock the following morning, as I could sleep no longer. The couple from Batavia was due at one o'clock. I decided to go uptown and get a cup of coffee and then returned home at about six. Connie was just getting up, as she couldn't sleep any longer either. We both sat down and had a cup of coffee with each other and talked about our upcoming move—we hoped. Connie then decided to go into the living room and watch TV for a while. I went outside to look around the grounds.

When I came in, it was ten thirty, and Connie was going to get into the shower. The phone rang just before she stepped in the shower. It was the people from Batavia wondering if they could come a little sooner to see the house again. They wanted to now stop by at noon, and I said okay. When Connie got out of the shower, I got in. I was out about eleven o'clock and got things ready for the couple stopping by the house. At ten minutes to twelve, the couple came to the door and rang the bell. I opened the door and greeted them with a hello and let them know we were glad they could stop by again.

The husband and wife asked if they could walk around the house by themselves for a few minutes, and then they had some questions. We had told them to take their time, and we would be ready to talk when they were. After about twenty minutes, they asked if we could sit down for a moment. We sat at the dining room table and offered them something to drink. They declined and then began asking their questions. We talked for about twenty minutes about the price and other things in the house. We finally came to an agreement, and they agreed to buy our home based on them getting a loan. They had to make a stop at a relative's house and would have the answer that afternoon.

They had to leave and said they would call us back that afternoon or the following morning. They thanked us for the chance to see the house again and were very excited about buying our home. They left, and we were so happy. We hoped that everything went okay.

CHAPTER 38

On May 22, 2007, we received a purchase contract for our house, and we immediately took it to our lawyer to put things in motion. The paperwork was finally in hand, and we had done it ourselves. We were so happy. Now everything was in full gear with us ready to sell the house. The people from Batavia liked the house and were very happy to buy it. The gentleman and his wife found exactly what they were after.

I also had to contact the moving company to get prices on moving everything to Arizona. Connie would be leaving on July 1 to meet Jen in Tucson. Due to my health regarding flying, I was staying behind and letting Connie fly to Arizona to pick out a home for us. I wish I could go, but I didn't want to take any chances of creating any problems when I would have to be traveling in a couple of months.

We had a meeting with the moving company on the twenty-first, and we went over everything to make sure all was covered. I also had to meet with the car carrier the following day to receive price quote on moving our car to Arizona. I would soon have all of the prices I needed for the move, and hopefully, all would go well.

The purchase contract had been approved by both parties, and the house would change hands in middle August for the house in Le Roy and also the one in Arizona I still had second thoughts about selling the house in Le Roy, but I didn't want to own all this property at once. I know that it would be okay.

In the next few weeks, Connie and I had a lot to take care of. We had the garage sale and sold the larger items in the house, such as the dining room table and the air compressor in the garage. I could not believe how good I felt, but I had to be very careful that I didn't overdo it. The move to Arizona was going to be a big one, and we had to be very careful.

I was very concerned about the trip. Sitting down for that long was really going to hurt me. I would have to really take it easy. I had started thinking about the move more and more. It was really a big thing we were doing. The big thing that really concerned me was that we had everything in Le Roy paid for, and now we would be getting into a large debt again. The thought of that really scared me. If something went wrong in Arizona, we could be in real trouble. But this whole thing was worth it if it made Connie happy. She truly deserved it after all she had put up with.

My back was still feeling really good with my new SCS. The device had given me a new life, which I never expected. I had my new life and the wife I love so much. I was so happy.

Connie and I wondered if we had everything covered. There is so much to do when you sell a house and move across the country. I had not been sleeping well lately thinking about all of the detail of our move. We had everything paid for, and now we would be starting all over again. Connie was worth every penny, as I owed my beautiful wife so much for all she'd had to put up with from me.

I would be taking her to the airport and sending her off to Arizona the following morning. We went to bed early and had to get up by seven o'clock. Connie's plane would leave at noon, and she had to be at the airport by ten.

We got up a little before seven. We had to shower and then get ready to leave. Connie had checked over the things she had packed to make sure she didn't forget anything. She'd had her shower and her coffee, and we talked a short time before leaving for the airport. On the way to the airport, we talked more about leaving for Arizona. We decided that this was something we really wanted to do. Jen was everything to us, and what would our lives be if we weren't able to see our baby? For the past six or seven years, I had not done anything because of my injuries. Connie had been watching me, so this was a good time to do something like this for us

With the spinal cord stimulator (SCS), my new life had begun. I never would have believed that I would have had a new chance at life. I thanked God every day for all he had done for me. I thanked Connie for standing beside me. So many times I thought of ending it all, and I was so glad that I didn't. There were so many things we had gotten through.

We arrived at the airport, and a skycap took Connie's bags out of the car. She went inside while I parked the car. When I got inside the terminal, she was ready to go to her gate, so I gave her a big kiss and hug. She then walked through security and vanished with all of the other people.

Her flight would take her about seven and a half hours. Jen would pick her up at the airport, and then Connie would be staying at Jen's house for the ten days she was there. Her schedule was to travel around with Jen while she could to look for a home for us. When Jen had to start work, Connie was going to travel with a realtor to look for a home.

We would talk on the phone every night. I knew she was really worried about me. As the week moved on, Connie found a house that she really liked. When Jen had time, Connie took her through it, and they both thought it was just terrific. Connie called me the night she had decided on the house she wanted. She was so excited and couldn't wait for me to see it. I told her if she liked it, to go ahead and sign the papers. The following day she sat with the realtor and signed the papers with the intent to buy. She called me when it was done to tell me.

Connie would be leaving for home in two days. I was glad she was so happy, as good things had not happened to Connie much since I'd been hurt in 2000. This was one big thing that would hopefully bring our marriage back together again.

I had treated her so rotten at times, but I realized that it was the pain talking. With this new SCS, I actually had a new life to where I could enjoy things and see people again. I couldn't wait to see the home she had picked out. I was sure it was beautiful. And I hoped it had a two-car garage!

CHAPTER 39

I tried to do things around the house while Connie was gone to help her out. Hopefully, when she got home she would be surprised and very happy about the work I'd done. The only problem I'd had while she was gone was overdoing it with my back. A couple of days I had to stay in and not go anywhere. I had to rest my back, so I spent time on the computer but only long enough to where I didn't hurt my back anymore. The ten days went by very quickly, as I tried to stay as busy as I could. I even went over to the neighbors and had dinner with them one night.

Connie was due back in two short days, and I would pick her up at the airport when she arrived. I was so happy that she was going to be home soon. I missed her very much. I did talk with her and Jenny on the phone several times, but it wasn't the same as having her home.

It was finally the day before Connie's homecoming. She had traveled around Green Valley, Arizona, as that's the location we'd picked out from looking at the map. Connie had found a nice home during the time she was in Arizona.

I was up at about eight o'clock the morning of July 17. I got ready and drove to the airport to pick Connie up at ten thirty. I waited for her to come up the ramp after getting off of the plane. I saw her in the distance, and as she got closer, I could see a big smile on her face. When she met me, she gave me a very big kiss and hug. I could tell that she was very glad to be home. I knew she was very tired, as she yawned a couple of times before we got to baggage claim to get her suitcase.

After getting her suitcase and taking it to the car, we talked about the great time she'd had in Arizona. She was very happy with the house she'd picked out for us and felt that we would have a good time living in Arizona and being close to our daughter. As I drove down the road, I could see that Connie had fallen asleep. She was obviously very tired, as she slept until we got home. When I pulled into the driveway, she finally woke up. She told me she was sorry for falling asleep, and I told her that she needed some rest. We got out of the car, retrieved the suitcases and small bags from the trunk, and took them into the house one at a time.

When we had everything in the house, Connie asked me if she could lie down for a short time. I told her to go ahead, and we would talk a little later. She went right into her bedroom and shut the door.

I had begun to think about when we bought our home in June 1968 and all the things we had done to it up to that point. We bought it for $16,000. We'd just gotten it the way we wanted it and then decided to sell it and move cross-country.

Our beautiful daughter was so important to us that we would go anywhere to be close to her. I knew that Connie couldn't be happier knowing that she would again be very close to Jen. All of this was well worth it.

The rest of July was quiet, and my back was still feeling good. Every day I woke up I couldn't believe that the pain was so much less than before the implant was done. I certainly hoped it would stay that way.

Connie and I worked around the house very hard to make sure everything was being taken care of. We would be leaving Le Roy for Arizona on August 16, 2007. I had to double-check with the moving company and car transport carrier to ensure everything was still on time. They were scheduled to be here on August 14 as we had agreed.

Our friends came to make sure that everything was taken care of and see if we needed more help. My back was still doing well with the spinal cord stimulator (SCS), and my new life appeared to be here for a long time. I was so happy that when we get to Arizona, I would be able to do more with Connie and Jenny. That is what I had been praying for more than six and a half years while I was dealing with intense pain.

When Connie woke up, it was two hours later. I knew that she was very tired and needed to get some rest. It was now four o'clock in the afternoon, and she felt refreshed to the point that she gave me a kiss. We sat down for a while so she could tell me about the house that she'd picked out. Everything sounded just great. I really couldn't wait to get to Arizona to see the house. I asked if she wanted something to eat, and she said maybe a little later.

My back had started to bother me a little more than usual, so I went into my room to turn the program up on my SCS. It took me about five minutes, and when I came out of my bedroom, Connie grabbed me and kissed me again. I asked her the reason for the kiss, and she said it was because of the work I had done in the house while she was gone. I had forgotten all about it.

CHAPTER 40

A few days had passed, and we were getting ready for the big move on August 14. It was now only four days away. Connie had gotten a phone call from one of our neighbors down the street to inform her that we were invited to a going away party at her house on the eleventh Ann and David were very good friends whom we had known for a long time. Connie thanked Ann for the call and hung up. When Connie told me, I kind of sniffled a little. It was going to be very hard to say good-bye to friends we had known for many years.

We had worked very hard around the house as we prepared to leave it behind and move to our new home in Arizona. Our next-door neighbors had come over a couple of times to help us out. We knew it was going to be very hard to say good-bye to them. We finally felt that everything was taken care of for the closing on our house. It would be very hard to leave the home that we'd had for more than forty years.

The going away party for us was the following day, and then the day after that, the movers would be here. Our trip would be on the fifteenth—just three days away. Things were moving so fast, and I hoped that we had covered everything. I had a few things to take care of in the garage, and I then would go into the house to rest for a while. While in the garage, I made the big mistake of picking up a garbage can that I'd forgot was full. I couldn't see it was full, because the top was on. When I bent over to pick it up, I really hurt my back. I didn't think it was too bad, but it hurt like hell. I began to think about the party and then the plane trip to Arizona on the fifteenth.

I took it easy for the rest of the day. I didn't tell Connie that I'd hurt my back, because I didn't want to give her something else to worry about. I took a hot shower and kept changing the programs on my SCS, which did help for a while. We had dinner, and I told Connie after dinner that I was tired and was going to bed early. She asked me if everything was all right, and I told her I was okay. I didn't like hiding things from her, but she had worried enough about me over the years. I wanted her to have a great day at the party the next night. I just hoped I could hide my pain from everyone.

I got up a couple of times during the night. The first time Connie still hadn't gone to bed, and she again asked me if I was all right. My back really was hurting me more than I had hoped. I changed programs again, but I could only have it so high while I was lying down. Although the stimulation was a little too strong for me while I was lying down, I did have it on that night. I hoped I could get to sleep again and also go to the party.

I had Vicodin to take if the pain became too strong. It had always helped me, as it was this time. I slept till about eight o'clock the next morning, and the party was in the afternoon. My back was still bothering me, but I thought I could make it through the party.

Connie and I had gotten ready and left the house a little before two o'clock. Ann and David only lived a couple of houses up the street. While walking to the house, we could see quite a few cars parked close by the house. As we walked beside the house, we could hear laughing in the backyard. My back was still hurting, but I knew I could make it through the party.

When we walked into the backyard, everyone began clapping. Connie and I both began to thank everyone for coming. About thirty people had showed up to the party, and it lasted about two hours. By the end, I could barely walk. The pain was very bad, and I really worried, as the movers would be at our house in the morning. I was fortunate enough to be able to get a ride home, as it was very painful to walk even that short distance. How was I going to deal with the movers tomorrow?

When I was taken home, Connie decided to walk. About five minutes after I'd returned home, she walked in the door and immediately asked what I had done to my back. The cat was now out of the bag. I told her how I'd hurt my back in the garage lifting a full garbage can and explained that the reason I didn't tell her was I didn't want to worry her. I told her I was going to call my rep from ANS/St Jude Medical in the morning to get an appointment to see him. He could come and hopefully reprogram my programmer so I could handle the pain much better than I was.

I had lived with this pain for so long, and at times, I wished I weren't even here any longer. I had created too much grief for everyone. I questioned whether it was worth it. My answer was no. I began to worry about my plane trip to Arizona. I feared the pain was going to be just awful, but I had better wait to see what happens.

The movers were on time. The car transport came on August 14, and I had to take the car to the old Continental Can building on Lake Street to load the car. The movers arrived at eight o'clock on the morning of the fourteenth and began loading all of our possessions. It took them seven hours to fully load the truck with everything. They told me they would be in Arizona on August 29 and no later unless something unseen had happened. We had to be at the airport at nine o'clock on the morning of the sixteenth, as our plane was leaving at eleven o'clock for Tucson. We did have a stopover at O'Hare Airport in Chicago for an hour, and then we'd be back en route to Tucson Airport.

I called my rep from ANS, and he agreed to meet me later on that day, as we were leaving the next morning. He did this as a huge favor to me. I couldn't thank him enough; at least I would have a new program to help me fight the pain. I had a friend of mine take me to my pain specialist in Rochester that afternoon to get my SCS reprogrammed.

Connie stayed home to handle the balance of the movers' job. Connie did a great job making sure all the things were loaded on the movers' truck.

After the reprogramming, I was on my way back home. When I got here, things were just great. Connie had everything covered, and the movers were all loaded and on their way to Arizona. Another friend of mine took our car to have it loaded on the car carrier, and the car would be there in about two weeks. Thank God for all of our friends, or we would not have been able to get both the movers and the car transport taken care of. Everything was done, and we would be leaving for Arizona the next day.

We made sure on the night of the fourteenth that we had everything covered. We had an early dinner and went to bed early. Our good friend was taking us to the airport, and we had to leave at eight o'clock in the morning. Both Connie and I went to bed at about nine and were up at six, so we could shower and get a quick bite to eat. We were picked up at eight o'clock on the nose and taken to the airport.

My back was feeling good. Once again, I thanked God for all of his help. The reprogramming worked out great. That had been the first time I needed help from my representative at ANS.

My wife was so happy, and she deserved everything she got. She had been my strength and had helped me through everything. She was quite a woman, and I loved her so much. She was so good to me.

I knew that Connie didn't like flying at all. We had been on airplanes together three different times, but she was still very fearful of not making it to our destination. We used to get flight insurance, because then Connie would at least feel that if anything happened to us, Jen would be taken care of. Connie missed Jen an awful lot, and I knew that being close to her would make Connie feel much better. This would be one of the things that I was able to do to pay Connie back for all the hell I had put her through. I had not been good to her, as the pain I lived with could really change a person a lot. No one, but no one, has any idea at all what chronic pain does to a person on the inside. Every minute of every day you feel that constant pain that travels throughout your body.

I was getting kind of anxious thinking about the house that Connie had picked out. I hoped that I would be able to do things around the house and enjoy the time we had together. I really thought that she picked out a beautiful home, and I couldn't wait to see it. We would be able to do a lot together with the help of my SCS.

I couldn't be luckier, and we would really begin to spend a lot of time together and maybe also have sex again. It had been more than seven years since Connie and I had even had a chance to lie next to each other. We had not spent any good time together since before I was hurt, and it might be because of me. I was afraid that I would hurt my back more. With the two steel rods implanted in my back, everything physical had stopped, and it was my fault.

Things definitely had to change so we could try to get back some of the life we'd lost. I was sure we would have to talk to a doctor about things before we jump into anything. I had to make a big effort, and then we could get some of our life back, I hoped. *With your help, God, we can do it together*, I prayed.

CHAPTER 41

Our flight took almost seven hours, and my back was very bad. Connie had given me a very strong pill on the way for relaxation, and I dozed off for most of the ride. When I did wake up, I was very groggy. When I moved around in the seat a little, I felt the pain go straight down my back. When we landed, it was very hard for me to stand up. When I stood to get into the wheelchair, the pain was very bad, and the tears rolled down my cheeks for a few seconds. No one could ever understand the very intense pain a person can have with a very bad back unless they go through it themselves.

I thought that things might have been different this time, but as usual, I was wrong again. I was really hoping that I could show the people that knew me that I'd finally come very close to beating this awful pain that I'd been living with for all these years. I had begun to cry, thinking that maybe I would have a life again, and my wife could lighten up with all of the things she had to do with me. How I loved my wife, and I wanted to repay her for all she did for me. She deserved everything I could give her and then more. I just hoped that I had the time to repay this most beautiful woman for all she had done. She had given her life to me doing everything I needed to try and live as comfortably as I could.

On the flight, Connie had been behind me all the time, making sure I was okay. She had a carry-on, and I had the larger of the two bags on my lap in the wheelchair. We had to go to the baggage claim to get our luggage and then go to get a car. When we went to baggage claim, at least I could take it easy for a while and relax a little with the pain I was going through.

I had to stand up so bad, and I finally had my chance. The aid held the chair while I stood up. I stood near the chair for about fifteen minutes and then began to walk around with my cane. It felt so good to be able to stand up and walk around a little, and my back began to loosen up. My back hurt quite a bit, and hopefully it would feel better after walking a little. It wasn't going to feel really good, but the pain level had dropped from about a ten-plus down to an eight or nine. After about fifteen minutes, we noticed the bag on the turnstile with our red yarn tied around the handle. I decided to walk to the car rental area, which wasn't far away.

We filled out all of the paperwork, and they brought the car up for us to get in. The car was not really big, but I could get my legs in and try to relax a little. We were leaving the Phoenix Airport and on our way to our new home. Connie drove about two hours and thirty minutes to Green Valley, Arizona, which was south of the airport. We pulled on to our new street, and Connie pointed it out to me. From the outside, it was a beautiful house. I couldn't believe it.

When I got out of the car, my back was very bad again. It took me time to stand up and then walk around in order for my back to loosen up before we could go into the house. Jen was already there and waiting for us. Connie had taken care of all of the paperwork during her trip out, but I would have to meet with the realtor the next day to finish signing some papers. In the meantime, we were still able to go in and look the house over. As we walked into the house, my back continued to hurt very badly, but I wanted to look around. The furniture and car would not be there for a couple of days, and we would have to stay in a motel until then.

We walked in the front door, and I was almost knocked over. What a beautiful house Connie had bought. I loved every part of it. It even had an electric fireplace, along with many other great things. My room was a big room off the back of the house with sliding doors that led to the Arizona room which is a screened in porch. It was just beautiful and also had a very large shower. I told Connie that I was very happy with everything about the house and complimented her that she couldn't have done a better job. She was so happy and put her arms around me and kissed me for quite a long time. It was by far the longest kiss I'd had from her in many months. I really knew now how happy she was, and that made me so happy. I loved her so much, and she was the love of my life. What a great day this was aside from all of the pain I had. The pain was well worth it. *Thank God for this great stimulator*, I thought. *This device really gave me a new life, which I never thought I would have again.*

Just before leaving the house, we received a phone call from the movers saying that they would not arrive for another three weeks. I was very mad when I got off of the phone and told Connie what the call was about. To stay in a motel for three weeks would cost us a fortune. My two sisters had winter homes in Arizona that were about an hour away. I decided to call my sister Sharon and tell her about out problem. She told us to go to Marana and stay there as long as we needed to. By now, my back was really bad. We had gotten directions from her and drove to Marana where the caretaker let us in.

What a lifesaver Sharon was. Sharon and Wayne had always been this kind. I was so proud to have such a wonderful sister with a great husband. They really saved us a lot of money by offering us their home in Marana. We would have to make sure that we reciprocated for the kindness they had extended to us.

It took us about an hour from door-to-door before we arrived at their home in Marana. When we arrived, I hit the bed as soon as we got in the door. My back was killing me, and I had to lie down right away. Connie had decided that she had to go and get some groceries, as there was nothing in the house to eat. We had past a supermarket just down the road, so she knew exactly where to go to get the groceries.

When Connie returned, I was out like a light. I was so tired from all the running around and the plane trip. We had to be in Green Valley at the realtor's office in the morning to sign the rest of the papers. I didn't know what time Connie had gone to bed, but I was there all night. I didn't eat until the next day. My back ached awfully when I got up. It was partly due to the bed I'd slept on, and the rest was due to the plane trip.

Connie and I both got ready, and we headed out to the realtor's office to sign the rest of the papers. With that, everything was done. Hurray! Eventually, with the stimulator and different programs I was able to use, my back began to feel much better. I was the luckiest man in the world to have found this brilliant device to take care of my back pain.

We were so lucky to have a place to stay before the movers arrived. Connie and I drove around Green Valley to see the different places and things the town had to offer us. Our house was centrally located with almost everything we needed in a two-mile radius—supermarkets, gas stations, a doctor's offices, a dentist, and many other things. There were people out near our home after we took ownership, and we met two neighbors who appeared to be very nice. Almost every day for close to two weeks we drove from Marana to Green Valley just to drive around.

Elaine and Sharon live in a community where the PGA played each year. It was a very nice place to live and very gorgeous with all of the mountains.

CHAPTER 42

Three weeks went by fairly quickly, and my back was feeling pretty good. And to top it off, the movers truck would be at the house the following morning. It took about six to seven hours to unload all of the items and set everything up as we needed. I had to lie down for about four hours because of my back. I really overdid it more than I should have, but things had to get done.

Jen came to the house in the morning to help us unload, and we were very happy to have her there helping. Thank God my SCS was still working fine. The device was a lifesaver to me, but when I overdid it, I had to pay for it the next day. We got the house set up the way we wanted it, and it really looked nice when we were done. We went to the different stores in town to get things we wanted to dress the house up to our taste.

We continued to put things where we wanted them. I couldn't get over how nice our new home was. Connie was so happy to have finally picked out the house of her dreams.

My back began to give me small problems, but I just figured that this was how the SCS worked. I never really searched out any possible problems, and honestly, I never thought to call the new rep here in Arizona. In fact, I hadn't even met my new representative. I just continued on doing anything that had to be done to get everything in place. Elaine had already come to her winter home in Marana, and Sharon wouldn't be here until after Christmas.

A month went by. It was September, and I started to really have problems with my SCS. I did have a local pain doctor who supposedly would work on them, but we had to talk to him about it. We make an appointment to see the doctor in Tucson and spend some time with him talking about the stimulator.

At our first meeting, he didn't seem too enthused with the SCS and said that we could get together at a later date. Connie and I had agreed when we got in the car that he was not the right doctor for me. I was not too impressed with how he felt about the SCS. It seemed as though he didn't want to be bothered with my problems. In essence, the SCS gave me a new life after all of the heavy pain I'd been subjected to. We really didn't know what to think after our first meeting with the doctor who was supposed to be really good with the SCS.

When I got home, I really worried what was going to happen to me if he didn't even suggest that I meet with the representative to see if we could determine what the problem was. I was not really thinking too straight with the pain drugs I was on, so I did nothing further. I felt that if the doctor thought I had a problem, he should have set me up with an appointment with some guys from ANS/St. Jude Medical.

At that point, I felt that I had a major problem and would never have the gift of less pain. I could not get out of my mind that things were not going to get any better with my unit, and I was truly going to suffer again for the rest of my life. I was beginning to make Connie's life hard, as the crying and hollering was taking over once again. What hell I put my beautiful wife through.

I pretty well gave up on my SCS, which had given me a new life for a very short time. I wondered why this would happen to me. I'd only had relief since May 2007 when it was put in.

Then I began to wonder why this hadn't happened before we moved. I felt that I was going to lose it out here with no help at all. Connie was here and enjoying being close to Jen, and I feared I would ruin it.

Connie and I talked and decided to go to a laser spine surgery seminar that was being offered in the foothills of Arizona. We thought it was worth looking into. Connie, in the meantime, continued to look into other doctors who may be able to help me. She worked very hard trying to get my life back to what it had been when the SCS was first put in. This lady has worked so hard for me, and I owe her so much for all she has done.

After thinking about the laser spine seminar, we became very interested. I was really wondering what they could do and what the cost may be to us. We had decided to go to the location and stay in a motel overnight. I was not really too excited, as I already knew what the SCS could do and was very impressed up until now.

We got ready for our trip to the foothills where this beautiful motel was and where the seminar would be held. Driving the roads through Tucson and to this big hotel was very scenic. As we got closer, we could see the building over the treetops and began to wonder how nice this place was. We finally pulled up in front of the motel, and it was absolutely beautiful. It was like something we had never seen before in our lives.

We parked the car, but getting out was a problem for me, as my back really hurt. I was going to have to walk around for a while to straighten out. After about ten minutes of walking, I felt better, and we went inside. Nothing was left to the imagination. It was so beautiful. We walked around a little and then made our way to the sign-in location. There were many people sitting down inside. I would have to let Connie sit, and I would stand up in back.

The seminar soon began and lasted about two hours. By the time it was over, my back and neck were killing me. I couldn't wait to get to the motel. The seminar was okay, but we would have to pay about $20,000, which was not totally covered by insurance. We were glad we'd gone and gotten information, but the SCS was still the only way to go.

Leaving this beautiful place was something we would never forget. It was so beautiful, and I thought maybe someday Connie and I could come here to stay a night.

We got into the car and drove to the hotel. I didn't even take my clothes off when we got into the room. I just crashed on to the bed and was out like a light and hurting an awful lot. Connie had stayed up for a while and then turned in herself. We were both up around seven o'clock the next morning and wanting to get coffee if possible. I walked to the checkout area and found a coffeepot. I got Connie a huge cup of coffee, which made her morning. She sipped it for a while, as it was very hot, and then she decided to take a shower. After she was done, we were on our way. I didn't want to take a shower there and would wait until we got home.

Several of our family members wanted to know about the seminar we'd gone to and wondered if it was a possibility for me. I had gotten in touch with Jen first and then my sisters to tell them it was a no-go. I wanted to continue with the SCS. I knew what type of feeling it could give me. All I have to do was find a doctor to help me with my problem. I didn't know how long it would take to find the right person to help me, but we would continue to look. Although we had discovered that the doctor we thought could help wasn't able to, we knew that was not the end.

I need to get that good feeling back that I'd had for such a short time. I was spoiled with the SCS, and it gave me a new life—something I never thought I would have in the beginning. I would not stop until I found a doctor who would help me. I realized the search may take us a long time, but we were hopeful that we could find a good doctor to help me. For the longest time, I suffered trying to search out a good pain doctor in Arizona. At that point, I was willing to go anywhere in Arizona to feel good again.

CHAPTER 43

It was February 2009, and it had taken nearly two years before we were able to find a doctor in Tucson. We were never able to figure out why we had been unable to find this doctor sooner. I had suffered with my back and neck pain for almost two years and even contemplated taking my own life a couple of times.

Connie had made an appointment to see the new doctor in Tucson the following week. My back and neck were giving me a lot of problems. It had been nine years since I'd fallen at work. The pain I have had to endure was so unbelievable for a person of this day to have to go through. I realized that the only way people may be able to understand was if I decided to write a book that detailed all of the things I had been through.

My appointment with Dr. W was scheduled for the following day at ten o'clock. Connie and I both went to bed early so we would hopefully be able to sleep. I didn't go to sleep right away and tossed and turned for quite a while. I finally fell asleep and woke up at six o'clock. I was really excited and hoping that this doctor could give me my life back. I prayed to God to please help me, as I could not continue like this much longer. I was so depressed and I hurt so badly that living the way I did was crazy. I wish that God would take me away from all of this. The pain was so bad now.

When I was done getting ready, we sat in the kitchen for a short time talking about this new doctor. Connie could see that I was very nervous and told me not to worry. She was so good like that, really worrying about me and how I felt. I loved her so much, and she was my whole life. Around eight thirty, we got in the car and left. Connie always liked the extra time, so we didn't have to hurry.

It took us forty-five minutes to get to the doctor's office. I was beginning to get a little nervous. We went to the second floor and found his office door. We walked in and saw the secretary, who asked us to sign in the book. She then instructed us to sit down and fill out some insurance papers. Connie always filled out the papers for me, so she got the papers and the clipboard, and she spent the next twenty minutes filling out all of the necessary pages. Shortly after we handed in the papers, a nurse came through a door and called out my name. We followed her into the doctor's office where she sat down with us and took some information from me. She took my blood pressure and weighed me and asked a couple of questions. Then she left the office.

About five minutes later, the doctor appeared through the office door and introduced himself to both of us. He then asked me why we were there to see him. I explained the problem I'd been having with my SCS, which I'd received in October 2007. I also told him about the other doctor we'd seen and relayed what he had told me. I could see in his face that he was a little put off by the comments the other doctor had made.

The doctor then explained that many things could happen to reduce the effectiveness of the stimulator. He questioned me about how the SCS was currently working. I told him exactly the feeling I was having and other different feelings I may have as the day went on. He suggested that the first thing that should be done was to have an x-ray of my back where the SCS was placed. After he got the x-rays and had a chance to review them, he would decide what should be done.

He wrote me a prescription to have my back x-rayed and instructed me to return to his office in two weeks. Connie and I thanked him and left his office. Before heading for home, we spoke to the receptionist and asked for an appointment to be made in two weeks. She gave us a card with the date on it, and we left the office ready to head for home.

When I got into the car, I told Connie that I was very impressed with this doctor. I could just tell that he was concerned and wanted to help me. Connie felt the same way. She started the car, and in forty-five minutes, we were home again. Connie told me that I should go to Carondelet Medical Group to have my x-ray done in the next couple of days. I wanted to have it done as soon as I could, so I went down to the medical center when I got up in the morning. It was about eight thirty when I walked through the door of the facility, and I noticed that quite a few people were already there. I waited about thirty-five minutes before I had the x-ray done. And then it took about thirty minutes once they finished all of the views that needed to be taken.

When we arrived home Connie had gotten a call to belong to a Mah Jongg group which played a very old chinese game. each week. Finally she is getting out.

CHAPTER 44

The two weeks until my next appointment seemed to go very slowly. My drug problem was really wearing on me, but there was nothing I could do but get through it. I did almost nothing for all of that time except to walk when I could. I really enjoyed taking walks during the day, as that was all of the exercise I would get. I needed to try to keep my weight down, as I knew being overweight was causing some of my problem.

Connie and I went to events at different places in Green Valley where people's wares were sold. She really enjoyed going to these outside functions, and I enjoyed it as well, as it kept us busy during some of our afternoons.

Before I knew it, I'd made it to the day before my follow-up appointment with the spine doctor in Tucson. Connie and I had dinner early and also decided to go to bed early.

I got up at about six thirty and turned the coffeepot on for Connie. She got up about seven, and we had to be at the doctor's office at ten o'clock. I was really excited and very nervous regarding the outcome of the x-rays. It seemed like Connie was taking all day to get ready. I was so excited at the thought that this doctor could help me with my problem.

Finally, Connie was ready at eight thirty, and we got in the car and left for Tucson. We pulled into the parking lot at quarter till and arrived at his office at ten o'clock sharp. The nurse came out to walk us to the doctor's office. Connie sat, and I began to pace as I always did, not being able to sit. We began to talk when the doctor walked in and wished us good morning.

We replied with the same, and then the doctor sat down and pulled the x-rays out of the large envelope.

He looked at my back and began to explain that there was something showing on the x-ray. He told Connie and me that it was probably scar tissue. He had run into this quite a few times while doing the implants and told me not to worry.

After we had talked about the scar tissue, he asked me if I was ready to get this over with and start to feel good again. I asked him how quickly he could do the procedure, and he said he could get me in for surgery the next week. We went ahead and scheduled the procedure for February 25, 2009, at nine o'clock in the morning.

I couldn't thank the doctor enough for the news he'd given me. Connie and I had to meet with the receptionist to get everything finalized, and then we left for home. The time felt like it was going slowly, as my back was really beginning to hurt a lot. The only good thing was that if this new SCS worked as good as the first one I'd had implanted, then I would be okay. I prayed to God that my back would be better after this new implant.

It had been seventeen months since I'd lost the stimulation in my first spinal cord stimulator (SCS). Having to relive the pain I'd experienced for more than seven years almost killed me more than once. Several times I had thought about suicide, and I didn't know why I never really did it. I guess that it was the love of my wife, daughter, and family all around me. Even my friends were very supportive. I have thanked God over and over again for helping me get through all the hard times. Finally, on February 25, 2009, I had gained a new life that was even better than the first SCS I'd had implanted. My new life was finally here again and better.

Time did go quicker than I had thought, and before I knew it, it was the day before I was to have the implant done. I had talked with my representative from St. Jude Medical, and he had high hopes of the outcome. I was feeling a little better thinking about this. I didn't know what Connie thought, as she didn't say much, but I was ready. I wasn't afraid at all but was positive that everything would work out fine.

Connie and I ate and then went to bed early so we could get up and get this all over with. It had been a long time since my stimulation had decreased, and I was happy that my relief would soon be here again.

We woke up around six o'clock the next morning, and I wanted to take my shower first, as I had a few things I wanted to do. I had been writing letters to God for the past eight years and telling him about the feelings I had. I felt that I could let him know both the good and bad things that were on my mind. I always thanked him for his help, and I always signed off with "I love you, God." This made me feel good that I could tell him my feelings.

Connie had taken her shower, and we had to be on the road by eight o'clock. It was now quarter till, and Connie made her coffee and put it into a special travel coffee mug. She really enjoyed her coffee during the day. I used to feel the same way until I'd been injured nine years earlier. For some reason, I just didn't drink it much anymore.

It took us forty-five minutes to get to the parking lot of the hospital, and we both stopped in the restrooms before entering the office. I'd said all of my prayers the night before, and I was confident that today was all set for me to become the happy disabled person I had tried to be for a long time. It was all in the doctor's hands now, and I had all the confidence in the world in him.

Connie and I walked up to his receptionist, and I signed in. Connie went and had a seat, and I paced as usual. I realized that it was bothering Connie today, as she looked very nervous. I felt real good and was looking forward to good things happening to me. We had waited about ten minutes before we were called into a special room where I changed into a gown. There was a bed in the room that I would lie on before going to surgery.

A nurse came through the door after I got dressed and started an IV solution that would gradually calm me down. The doctor joined us before we were to go into surgery to explain a couple of things to Connie and me. The doctor was very nice and really cared about his patients, which was the way my first doctor should have been a couple of years earlier. I really felt at ease with this doctor. He told us about the procedure and then he left for the surgery room.

The nurse who was standing in the room walked over and gave me a shot before we left, and I began to feel just a little funny. I kissed Connie before they took me away, and when I reached the surgery room, I was given another shot. They asked me to count backward from one hundred. I had to remain just slightly awake, as the doctor would be asking me questions regarding the location of the bad nerves in my back.

The surgery took about two and a half hours because the doctor had to remove the scar tissue from my previous operations. We were told there would be increased swelling around the area where he had to remove the scar tissue. After surgery, I was taken to the recovery room to completely wake up from anesthesia. The spotting of the wires was also completed, but there was going to be swelling due to the removal of the scar tissue.

I was eventually taken to my room where Connie was waiting for me. Connie greeted me, and I am sure she was glad that this was finally over with after waiting almost two years to get a new SCS. About ten minutes after I'd arrived back in my room, the doctor came in to tell us that everything went well. He said I should have great stimulation to my back and neck area and then told us that the representative from St. Jude would be in to program my generator, which was implanted in my buttock area.

Just as the doctor finished talking to us, the man from St. Jude walked through the door. He had me stand up so he could do the programming, and about ten minutes later, he had me turn on my unit. I felt instant stimulation, and I was so happy. I looked over at Connie, and she was crying a little. I knew that I finally had made it. My new life began on February 25, 2009, and we now would begin to enjoy life again together.

CHAPTER 45

With my new start on life, Connie and I were able to get out more and have lunches again at restaurants. I just had to be sure to bring my large gel pillow to sit on in case we didn't get a booth. We began to do more and more small things together, and Connie really seemed to be enjoying the new me more each day.

On occasion, I needed to have my SCS adjusted when my back hurt a lot, and the stimulator wasn't handling the pain well. The representative would come to the hospital or my doctor's office in Green Valley and input new programs into my controller. The whole process would take about thirty minutes, and then I would be good to go. The new SCS was a godsend.

After the problems I'd had with my first SCS from October 2007, I'd had to wait two years for my new SCS. It had, once again, given me the new life I had been praying for since the first unit stopped working. Many times before getting the new implant, I had considered ending my life and taking the pressure off of Connie. I was so glad that God had intervened and convinced me that giving up was not the right thing to do. We had faced so many hardships since I'd been hurt, but with Connie's help, we were able to get through them.

Things were going much better for us until March 2009 when, once again, we had to face a very bad problem. I had been on the fentanyl patch for almost seven years for my intense pain. With the new SCS, my pain was reduced by 50 percent. The fentanyl patch cut another 30 percent of my pain, and I had Vicodin for any additional pain when I needed it.

One day in March I went to the pharmacy to take in my prescription for the fentanyl patch, which I needed for that month. I left the prescription and told the associate that I would return the following morning to pick up the medication. When I returned the following day, I was advised that the price on the medication had changed from a $7 monthly co-pay to a $95.20 monthly co-pay. I almost fell over on the floor, as I could not believe what I was hearing. I went right home and told Connie what had happened. She didn't believe it and went to get the booklet from AARP, which lists drug prices. She did find something, but it wasn't clear to me, so she called AARP and they confirmed the price was correct. Connie had asked how long the new price would be in effect , and she was told that they were not sure at this point..

We could not believe this big problem. It seemed to just one thing after another for us. Unfortunately, we didn't have a lot of money due to the due to the outcome of the lawsuit but we would get through this somehow, just as we had with everything else. The amount of money I received was very small compared to me living like this for the rest of my life. I had realized to late that it should have never been settled until a later date depending on my condition. Ever since I'd been hurt, I had dragged our family down with regard to everything. When we lived back East, we owned everything and had a good nest egg, which we had to use after my accident.

Once we learned of the drastic cost increase for the patches, Connie called our family doctor's office to make an appointment to see him about my drug problem. I thought of the thousands of other people who were also on the fentanyl patch and what they were facing now. The drug companies were getting rich, and everyone else was going broke.

We got in to see my doctor and presented my problem to him. He couldn't believe what was happening to me again. He nicely said that I had been through enough without having to deal with this problem. He had read that there was going to be an increase, but he couldn't remember how much. He told me that he would put me on morphine sulfate, but I would have to get all of the fentanyl out of my system before it could be determined how much morphine I would need to deal with my pain. He warned me that it was going to be rough on me for a while. What else was new? He started me out on a small dosage and would have to work me up. It was going to take a few months before I would finally make the changeover.

It was now late October 2009, and I had been having a very rough time during the changeover. Between the pain in my back and neck and also the drug transition, I was really suffering at times. I began to get depressed going through all of this crap. And there was no one to help me, as I was the one going through all of this.

Connie, Jen, and my sisters felt so bad for me having to live through this very difficult time in my life, as if I hadn't been through enough already. The day now was the early morning of October 30, 2009, and I was very depressed with all of these problems I was facing. The transition was not complete, and I had finally had it. I just couldn't handle it anymore. I began making a plan to kill myself that day. I just had to figure out how and where.

I began to pace back and forth on our patio, and that continued for about half an hour when Connie was up and walked through the sliding doors. She said good morning to me. I replied the same to her but in a very low voice. She knew right away that there was a problem with me. She didn't say much for about five minutes, and then she asked me what was wrong. I replied nothing and then told her I was going to take a walk. She said okay, and I left.

I had walked around the subdivision thinking about how I was going to kill myself. I'd finally had enough of the pain and the problems I'd faced every single day since October 3, 2000. I had put Connie through hell with no real end in sight.

One of the big problems I had was that I had two large life insurance policies, and if I just killed myself, Connie would not get the benefits of the two policies. To ensure she'd be taken care of, I would have to do something that wouldn't be an obvious suicide to the insurance companies.

I had made my mind up that I would do it either later that day or that night.

I returned home, and Connie asked me to sit down and talk with her. I told her that I didn't want to talk, and I was going into the bedroom to listen to the radio. It was now twelve thirty in the afternoon, and I decided to turn the TV on to watch something while I was planning to end my life.

I woke after two hours of sleep and began crying quietly, remembering that I'd had enough of all the pain and shit in my life. I went out into the kitchen to get a drink, and Connie was sleeping on the couch but quickly woke up when she heard me in the kitchen. She again asked me to sit down and talk with her, and again, I told her I didn't want to. When I closed my bedroom door, I could hear Connie crying, trying to keep it very low. With the way I felt, her crying didn't faze me. Had I not been so badly depressed, I would have been in the living room in a flash. But in the moment, I had few feelings for anyone.

About seven years earlier, I'd ended up at a hospital in Rochester, New York, for depression, and they fed me with different drugs. I didn't want any drugs, as I wanted to make sure I did it in a way that no one would know it was intentional. I watched TV and went to the bathroom. I could hear Connie sniffling.

I had decided that I was going to do it in the car. But how would I do it so no one would be the wiser? I kept thinking about it until I fell asleep. I hadn't slept well the night before, so I was out like a light for the rest of the night. When I awoke at about six thirty the next morning, I felt great. I hadn't yet thought about my plans of the day before. When it did come to me, I couldn't believe that I felt so good this morning. I got up and walked out into the living room, and it was quiet and still a little dark out. I looked into Connie's room, and she was sleeping quietly in bed. I still could not believe that I felt so good, especially when I was ready to kill myself less than twenty-four hours earlier. What had happened to me? I had no idea at all and still couldn't believe it.

I decided to get dressed and then take a ride in the car, as I didn't want to make any noises to wake Connie up. I felt so bad about how I'd treated her the day before. I was rotten to her and made her cry and everything. Why had I done all of that? What was wrong with me?

I got into the car and backed it out of the driveway and then just drove around Green Valley with no intention of really going anywhere. After driving for about forty-five minutes, I decided to go to the department store, which was open all night. I walked in at about seven thirty and just walked around for a while. Thinking about everything that happened the day before, I realized that I must have really upset Connie, and I felt so bad. Even though I felt great today, she didn't know what to think or what I was thinking. This was how I had treated her since I'd been hurt almost nine years earlier. I loved her so much, but I had also put her through so much hell. She had stuck by me every single day, and things like this happened.

I got into the car at about eight fifteen and drove home. Connie was still sleeping, so I thought I would get on the computer. I turned it on and then began to surf the web. One of my classmates had put a general note to all of our graduating class members. It said: "I was notified this morning David Orlando died during the night in Florida."

When I read that, a big surge went up to my brain. I couldn't believe it. I was devastated by the news. David and I had been very close friends for many years. We would call each other, and when we lived back East, he would come to my home and visit or go to my mom's to visit. He was actually another member of our family.

I had been trying to contact him for the past six months. I sent him letters and called him to no avail. I thought that he was mad at me for some reason. I couldn't believe that he was gone. I loved David Orlando. Then it hit me! This was why I woke up that morning feeling so good. David had given his life for me, so I wouldn't kill myself and leave Connie and Jenny alone. I kept saying to myself, *Thank you, David. Thank you, David.* David had saved my life, and I loved him so much for giving his life for mine.

Thank you, David, for everything, my brother, I thought. *I love you very much.*

This was another very hurtful thing in my life. I couldn't help but wonder when all of this was going to stop. I'd had enough and wanted no more, please. Connie and I had been through so much in our lives, and I just prayed that we were done with all of the crap we'd had to put up with over the years.

Connie had walked into the kitchen and saw me in my bedroom on the computer. When she walked into my room I had given her the news and explained what had happened to me.

CHAPTER 46

Two years had gone by, and my life was just great. I still lived with pain every minute of every day, but it was manageable with my SCS. I had received a new life from my new implant on February 25, 2009. The drug issue was also over with, and I was now on 360 milligrams of morphine sulfate a day for my pain. I lived with pain every minute of every day, but the huge difference was that it was manageable. I was able to live a fairly close to normal life with my spinal cord stimulator (SCS). I sometimes thought about where I would have been today had I not taken the trial test. Probably dead.

In April 2011, Connie began to feel really bad. This was the beginning of the end for my beautiful and most loving wife of more than forty-five years. She was diagnosed with lung cancer and eventually died on February 25, 2012, just three years after my latest spinal cord stimulator (SCS) implant. She was my whole life, and she was so happy moving to Arizona to be with her beautiful daughter, Jen. It was a true honor to have married Connie Lee Chiler on August 27, 1966, in a small church wedding in Le Roy, New York. She was the most loving and kindest woman I had ever known. God Bless you, my one and only wife. I love you so much.

With the loss of Connie, my life was turned upside down. We had been together for so long and had gone through many ups and downs in our lives. We enjoyed each other so much and dedicated our lives to our very special daughter. She had made us so happy with all of her accomplishments. Now, with Connie gone, I had no idea what I was going to do with my life. I have very few friends here in Arizona and belong to no organizations. I have thought about this quite a bit, and I found myself very lonely in the beautiful house she had picked out. I have thought about leaving here, but Connie made me promise to take care of Jen. I wonder at times who is going to take care of me.

My sisters have been a very big help to me. I know that my head is not on straight, and my pain is up and down. Many times, I forget to turn up my SCS when the pain becomes really bad. I have tried to be strong for Jen, but it has been very hard for me due to the closeness Connie and I shared. I am trying my best to stay in close contact with Jen, and I am very glad that she has very close friends at work.

I try very hard to keep busy around the house. Unfortunately, I overdo it quite a bit and then have to live with a lot of pain the next few days, depending how bad I overdid it. I was taking more Vicodin than usual just to get me through the days. I tried to make a list of things that I have to do and then work the list down. This lasted for a couple of weeks before I decided to try visiting the local nursing home.

I had called there to speak with someone who could tell me what I had to do to visit with some people there. I talked with a lady who told me just to stop by and ask for her, and she would meet with me to go over what I could do. I waited for a couple of days and then drove there to meet with her. I parked out front of the home and walked through the front door. There was no one at the front desk. I stood there for about ten minutes, but still, no one showed up to greet me. I decided to walk around the corner and saw a person in the office who asked what I was after. I explained that I was there to see Joan about visiting some of the patients there. The woman told me that Joan was not in on that day and suggested that I call the next time before I came.

About a month and a half had passed since Connie's death when I received a call from an in-home nursing company that had taken care of Connie. They were going to send me a grief counselor if I was interested in seeing one. I told them that I would like to have someone come by so I could talk to him. About two days later, a man stopped by, and we chatted for an hour about things that were going on in my mind. Before he was ready to leave, we set a date for the following week. This began to make me feel a little better, talking about all of the problems I had to deal with.

As the time went by, my back and neck were pretty good some days, and other days I felt the pain of overdoing it. I could not get used to not trying to work so hard around the house. When my sisters came on Sundays, they would tell me the same thing.

The grief counselor came for about six months before he got sick and was no longer able to schedule appointments. I liked him a lot, and now I would have to start over with someone else. Finally, a young lady showed up at the door and introduced herself as Jennifer. She was very nice and had lived back East as I had. She continued to come to the house for another six months. Then the time came when she was all through. I had the two individuals for a total of one year, and I hadn't had to pay for their services. They really helped me very much, and I really appreciated their concern for me.

In July 2013, I decided to travel back East to visit my hometown. I was made an honorary member of the class of 1963, which was Connie's graduating class. They were having their fiftieth reunion, and I decided to go home and attend. This would be the first trip that I would make by myself, and I have to say that I was a bit scared. I had all my medications, and I would take one very strong pill that would almost knock me out due to the tremendous pain I would incur riding that far. It was difficult for me to sit a long time without getting up to stretch and walk around so my back wouldn't cramp up. I had made it to the airport in Rochester, New York, after a seven-hour plane ride, and I was a complete mess. I had a good friend of mine pick me up at the airport and take me to the motel near my hometown.

When I arrived at the motel, my friend helped me in with my bags and then left, as I had to lie down for a long time to hopefully straighten up before morning. I was up several times during the night. When I finally got up in the morning, my back really hurt. I took my normal pills first thing in the morning, and then I also took a Vicodin for the additional pain. I called the car rental place, and they were coming to pick me up at ten o'clock. I had two hours to get ready, and then after I got the car, I would drive to my hometown.

I was ready to go when the man from Enterprise picked me up. We then had to drive back to the rental office, so I could sign all of the papers. When I was done, I was off to Le Roy. I got there at about noon and drove right to my friend's house to say hello. I spent a short time there and then traveled to the next stop. Unfortunately, while I was home, I really overdid it and never made it to the reunion, which was the entire reason I had gone home.

I had made so many stops that I ended up in my motel four days sooner than I wanted. I spent most of my time in bed trying to get my health back to where it should be. I was home for ten days and ended up lying in bed for four days. I really made a very big mistake. I vowed that this would never happen to me again.

I left New York on a Tuesday headed for Tucson and arrived home almost nine hours later. My back, once again, was very bad. My daughter picked me up at the airport and took me home. My class reunion is in 2014, so I hope to travel back to Le Roy again that summer.

After getting home, I relaxed for about two weeks without doing anything too strenuous.

I got up one morning in late August 2013 and decided to go to the casino, as I began to get very lonely with no one in the house but me. That one day began a daily trip to the casino. I eventually met almost all of the employees at the casino to where they have started calling me Scotty when they see me in the morning.

Due to my poor sleeping habits, I will go to the casino any time between eleven o'clock at night and six o'clock in the morning. It is exactly nine miles north of my house on the way to Tucson. I found that I really enjoy going to the casino as long as I don't lose. I only take about sixty dollars with me, and hopefully, I end up making enough to prevent me from taking a lot of money out of my savings account. The casino serves excellent food, but I seldom get any. At times, I wish that I could stay home in bed rather than going to the casino. When I decide to cool it for a while, I change my mind and go anyway.

During the first week of November 2013, I received a letter from United Healthcare indicating that they were going to cut my intake of morphine from six pills a day to four pills a day. If this would not be possible, my doctor had to write an exception letter to Untied Healthcare, which he did.

A month went by, and I hadn't heard anything from my doctor or United Healthcare. I had something else to inquire about, so I decided I would also ask about my morphine exception letter. After taking care of the first problem, I asked about my morphine exception. The individual I was talking with looked into the computer and advised me that I had been denied. I almost fell to the floor. I couldn't believe this, as I had been on this morphine for more than three years.

In fact, I had to transition off of the fentanyl patch due to the cost to begin taking the morphine sulfate. The person on the phone told me that they had not received the information from my doctor soon enough. In fact, they didn't even show that he had replied at all. As soon as I was done with United Healthcare, I immediately called my doctor's office. I explained my problem, and his nurse told me that she would call me back. She called me back about an hour later and told me that they had replied to the letter in December 2013. I didn't know what to do then. I thanked her and hung up.

My God above must have been listening, as a little later I went out to get the mail and received a leaflet in the mail saying that Congressman Ron Barber would be in town the upcoming Saturday to great residents of Green Valley. I had figured that I had nothing to lose, so I wrote it on the calendar to be at the supermarket where he would be and try to talk to him.

During the next few days, I had done nothing but go to the casino and look at the walls of my house by myself. When Saturday came, I was up at about four o'clock in the morning and went to the casino. I was there for about three hours and returned home at about seven. When I got home, I had something to eat, and then I wanted to take a shower. After the shower, I got on to the computer for a couple of hours until it was time to leave.

The supermarket was only five minutes from my house, and I arrived a little early. The chairs were lined up along the outside wall. They were fold-up chairs, and there was no way I could sit on one of them. That was okay anyway, as they were all taken. I had to walk back and forth so my back wouldn't cramp up on me. The congressman wasn't there yet, but after walking back and forth for about thirty minutes, a lady who was first in line walked back to me and asked if I would like to go to the head of the line and talk to the congressman first. I thanked her very much and gladly walked to the front of the line.

Just a few minutes later, Congressman Ron Barber walked toward me from the road and put his hand out and shook mine. He asked me what he could do for me, and I explained about my problem with no longer getting enough morphine for my pain. I told him what had happened over the last month and a half, and he told me that his staff would look into it on Monday. He asked me to walk over with his staff member to give her the information she would need to look into my problem on Monday. I gave her ID numbers and answered other questions she had. When we were done, I thanked her for everything and walked to my car.

I truthfully did not expect anything to happen and worried about my upcoming transition during the whole weekend. On Tuesday of the following week, I received a phone call from United Healthcare regarding my denial. The lady who called had told me that Congressman Ron Barber's office had called and wanted them to reexamine the denial letter I had received in the mail. The lady said that she would call me back in a day or two.

A day later she called back and asked me to call the AARP Pharmacy and give them my name, and they would know what to do. As soon as our call ended, I called the number she had given me. When a lady answered, I told her my name and that I was supposed to call her. She asked me what for, and I explained that all I was told to do was to give her my name. She told me she knew nothing about me. We ended the call, and I called the lady from United Healthcare again, telling her that the lady knew nothing about me.

The woman from United Healthcare said that she would call me back in an hour or two. She called back in an hour and told me that the denial had been reversed, and I was approved to take six morphine pills a day. I was so happy, but I wouldn't believe it until I got it in writing. Two days later, I received a letter from Congressman Barber's office with a copy of the letter from Untied Healthcare advising that the denial had been reversed and I would receive six pills a day.

I thanked my God for the help he sent to me. I have been very fortunate in the past couple of years since my wife passed away. I have had my family and my God above to take care of me. With this book, I hope that many people are able to get a handle on the pain they live with today and get direction on how to get the relief that they desperately need. God bless you all.

My Special Salute to All Sufferers of Chronic Pain

I am one of the few people in the world today who knows what you have to deal with every day. The only thing I don't know is the type of pain you are dealing with. I can tell you that there are things being discovered every day to help people with all kinds of pain. Do not lose hope. Keep in very close contact with your pain specialist, because he has the knowledge of what is available to possibly help you.

God bless all of you!

Family Members Who Passed Away and a Very Close Brother of Mine (Adopted)

Connie Chiler Scott, wife, passed away in February 2012
David Orlando, brother, passed away in October 2009
Rose B. Scott, mother, passed away in December 2006
Willis G. Scott, father, passed away in June 1985
Rozella Scott Stone, sister, passed away in September 2001
Edward Stone, brother-in-law, passed away in March 2004
Jerry Stone, nephew, passed away in June 2005
Shirley Scott Lathan, cousin, passed away in March 2012

Letter to Normals

I would like to state that this "Letter to Normals" be used to help other people with FMS as long as proper credit is given to Bek Oberin (Bek wrote the "Open Letter to Those without CFIDS"). This letter was modified (with permission) and published by Paula Payne in 1996 to become the "Letter to Normals."

Letter to Normals from a Person in Chronic Pain:

Having chronic pain means many things change, and a lot of them are invisible. Unlike having cancer or being hurt in an accident, most people do not understand even a little about chronic pain and its effects, and of those they think they know, many are actually misinformed.

In the spirit of informing those who wish to understand:

These are the things that I would like you to understand about me before you judge me.

Please understand that being sick doesn't mean I'm not still a human being. I have to spend most of my day in considerable pain and exhaustion, and you visit, sometimes I probably don't seem like much fun to be with, but I am still me, stuck inside this body. I still worry about school, my family, my friends, and most of the time, I'd still like to hear you talk about yours, too.

Please understand the difference between "happy" and "healthy." When you've got the flu, you probably feel miserable with it, but I've been sick for years. I can't be miserable all the time. In fact, I work hard at not being miserable. So, if you're talking to me and I sound happy, it means I'm happy that's all. It doesn't mean that I'm not in a lot of pain, or extremely tired, or that I'm getting better, or any of those things. Please don't say, "Oh you're sounding better!" or

"But you look so healthy!" I am merely coping. I am sounding happy and trying to look normal. If you want to comment on that, you're welcome.

Please understand that being able to stand up for ten minutes doesn't necessarily mean that I can stand up for twenty minutes or an hour. Just because I managed to stand up for thirty minutes yesterday doesn't mean that I can do the same today. With a lot of diseases you're either paralyzed, or you can move. With this one, it gets more confusing every day. It can be like a yo-yo. I never know from day to day, how I am going to feel when I wake up. In most cases, I never know from minute to minute. That is one of the hardest and most frustrating components of chronic pain.

Please repeat the above paragraph substituting "sitting", "walking", "thinking", "concentrating", "being sociable" and so on, it applies to everything. That's what chronic pain does to you.

Please understand that chronic pain is variable. It's quite possible (for many, it's common) that one day I am able to walk to the park and back, while the next day I'll have trouble getting to the next room. Please don't attack me when I'm ill by saying "But you did it before!" or "Oh, come on, I know you can do this!" If you want me to do something, then ask if I can. In a similar vein, I may need to cancel a previous commitment at the last minute. If this happens, please do not take it personally. If you are able, please try to always remember how very lucky you are, to be physically able to do all of the things that you can do.

Please understand that "getting out and doing things" does not make me feel better, and can often make me seriously worse. You don't know what I go through or how I suffer in my own private time. Telling me that I need to exercise, or do some things to "get my mind off of it", may frustrate me to tears, and is not correct, if I was capable of doing some things any or all of the time, don't you know that I would? I am working with my doctors and I am doing what I am doing what I am supposed to do. Another statement that hurts is, "You just need to push yourself more, try harder". Obviously, chronic pain can deal with the whole body, or be localized to specific areas. Sometimes participating in a single activity for a short or a long period of time can cause more damage and physical pain than you could ever imagine. Not to mention the recovery time, which can be intense. You can't always read it on my face or in my body language. Also, chronic pain may cause secondary depression (wouldn't you get depressed and down if you were hurting constantly for months or years?), but it is not created by depression.

Please understand that if I say I have to sit down, lie down, stay in bed, or take these pills now, that probably means that I have to do it right now, it can't be put off or forgotten just because I'm somewhere, or I'm somewhere, or I'm right in the middle of doing something. Chronic pain does not forgive, nor does it wait for anyone.

If you want to suggest a cure to me, please don't. It's not because I don't appreciate the thought, and it's not because I don't want to get well. Lord knows that isn't true. In all likelihood, if you've heard of it or tried it, so have I. In some cases, I have been made sicker, not better. This can involve side effects of allergic reactions, as in the case with herbal remedies. It also includes failure, which in and of itself can make me feel even lower. If there were something that cured, or even helped people with my form of chronic pain, then we'd know about it. There is a worldwide networking (both on and off the Internet) between people with chronic pain. If something worked, we would KNOW. It's definitely not for lack of trying. If, after reading this, you still feel the need to suggest a cure, then so be it. I may take what you said and discuss it with my doctor.

If I seem touchy, it's probably because I am. It's not how I try to be. As a matter of fact, I try very hard to be normal. I hope you will try to understand. I have been, and am still, going through a lot. Chronic pain is hard for you to understand unless you have had it. It wreaks havoc on the body and the mind. It is exhausting and exasperating. Almost all the time, I know I am doing the best to cope with this, and I live my life to the best of my ability. I ask you to bear with me, and accept me as I am. I know that you cannot literally understand my situation unless you have been in my shoes, but as much as is possible, I am asking you to try to be understanding in general.

In many ways I depend on you, people who are not sick. I need you to visit me when I am too sick to go out. Sometimes I need you to help me with the shopping, the cooking or the cleaning. I may need you to take me to the doctor, or the store. You are my link to the "normalcy" of life. You can help me to keep in touch with the parts of life that I miss and fully intend to undertake again, just as soon as I am able.

I know that I asked a lot from you, and I do thank you for listening. It really does mean a lot.

I wish you all good luck, and make sure that you give one of these letters to each of your family members and friends so they truly know what you are going through. It was the best thing I did, as I found that no one really knew or understood everything I was going through.

Richard N. Scott

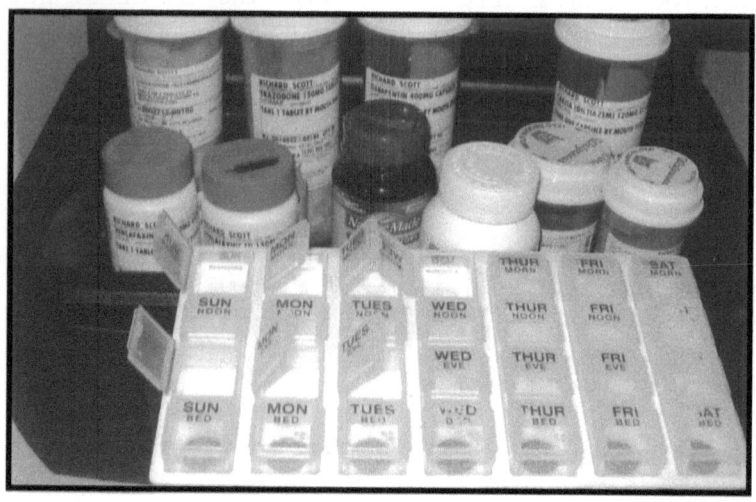

Current List of Drugs Taken by Richard N. Scott (DOB 9/30/45)

Effexor XR	150 mg	1 tablet in p.m.
Hydrocodone/APAP	10/750T changed 10/28/13	3 to 4 tablets a day as required
Lorazepam	.05 mg	2 to 3 daily as needed for anxiety
Gabapentin	400 mg	1 capsule in a.m.; 1 capsule in p.m.
Morphine Sulfate ER	60 mg	3 tablets in a.m.; 3 tablets in p.m. Total Daily Dose 360 mg
Fenofibrate 160 mg	**Removed by DR. Ata on 8/1/13**	**1 tablet in p.m.**
NITROSTAT	.04 mg tablets 25's	as needed
ASA	81 mg	1 tablet in p.m.
Diltiazem SR (Cartia XT)		1 tablet in p.m.
Mineral Oil		1 tablespoon every other day or as required

D3 5000 TS   1 tablet in p.m.

Allergic To: Nubain-Dilaudid-Silfa

My drug log is used to record my daily intake of drugs.

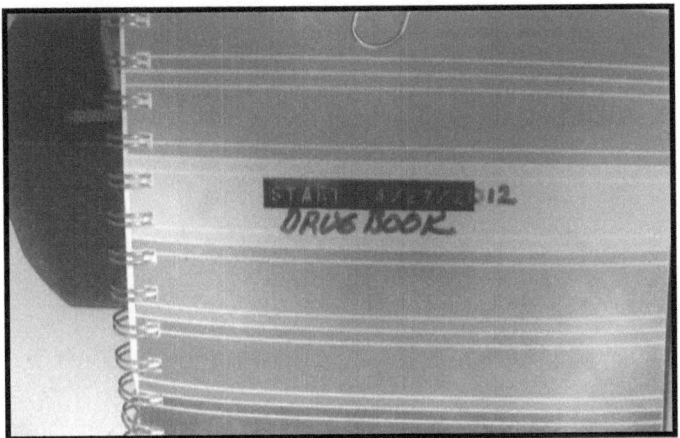

233

SUMMARY

In October 2000, I was injured by a very serious fall down a concrete and steel staircase. I lived through constant hell with the strongest pain I'd ever had. At times, I had thoughts about taking my own life, but my wife and I worked hard at taking one day at a time. I had two surgeries, which both failed. I had seen many doctors and taken many medications to reduce the pain. There were times when I lived like a zombie due to the strength of the medications I was taking. Finally, that day I prayed for—the chance to change my life forever—came.

TENS Unit

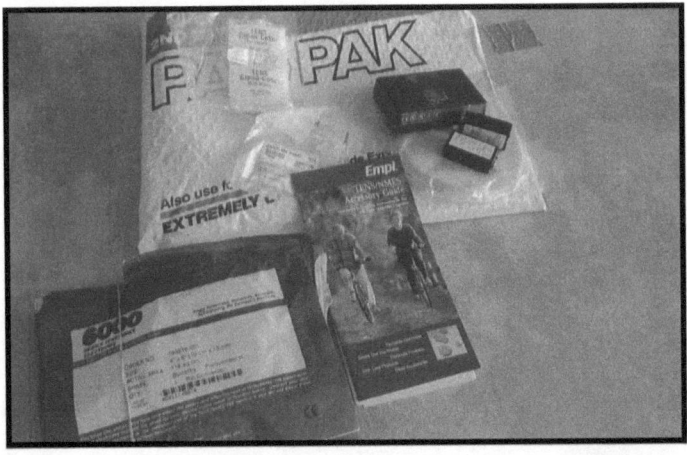

A TENS unit treats many kinds of pain. It can help lessen acute (short-term) pain like after surgery or an accident. TENS lessens pain by sending painless impulses through electrodes (sticky patches) placed on the skin.

The electrical signals travel from the TENS unit, through wires, and to the electrodes.

Plastic Back Brace

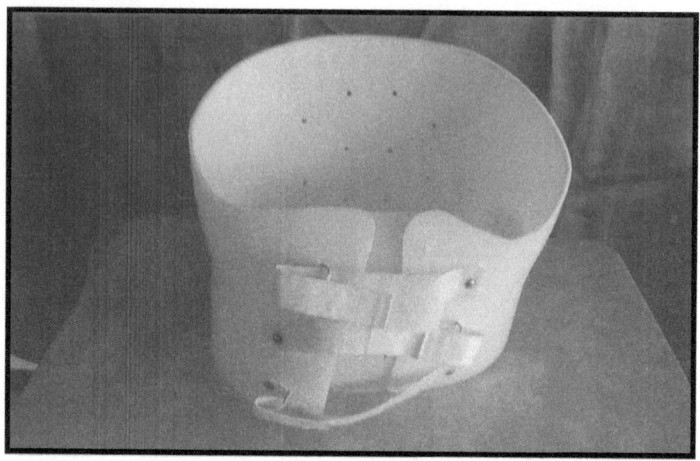

This was the first brace I used after my surgery in New York.

The Miami J Cervical Collar

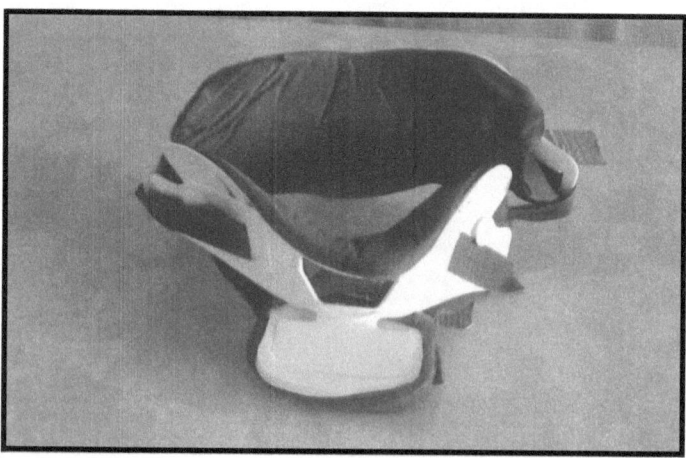

The function of this brace is to keep your neck immobilized, to decrease pain, and to allow your injury to heal. Some of your normal daily activities may be restricted due to this type of collar.

Spinal Fusion System

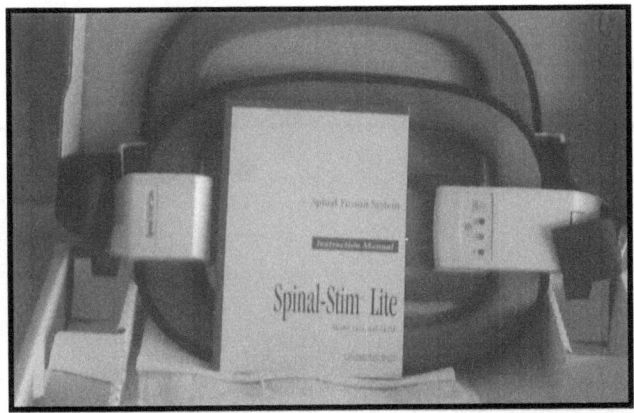

Spinal-Stim is a noninvasive, electromagnetic bone growth stimulator indicated as a spinal fusion adjunct to increase the probability of fusion success and as a nonoperative treatment or salvage of failed spinal fusion, where a minimum of nine months has elapsed since the last surgery. The system is recommended for daily application, at least two hours per day, for a minimum of ninety days to a maximum of two hundred seventy days.

ORTHOFIX Physio-Stim Lite Bone Growth Stimulator

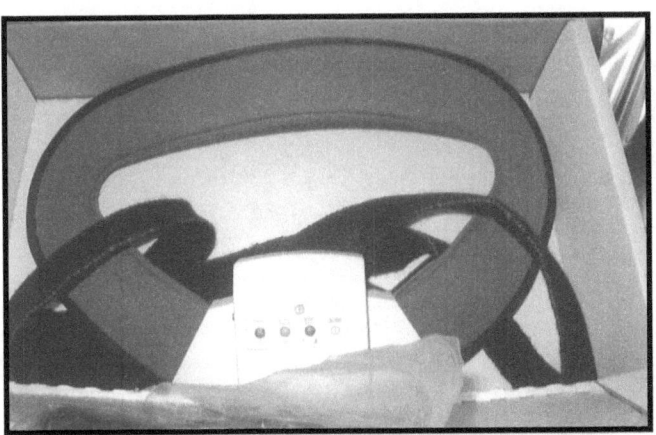

The Spinal Stim spinal fusion system is a safe nonsurgical treatment your doctor has perscribed to aide the healing of your spinal fusion. Spinal

Stim is a bone growth stimulator which uses a very low- strength pulsed electromagnetic field (PEMF) to activate the body's natural healing process.

Orthotrac Pneumatic Vest

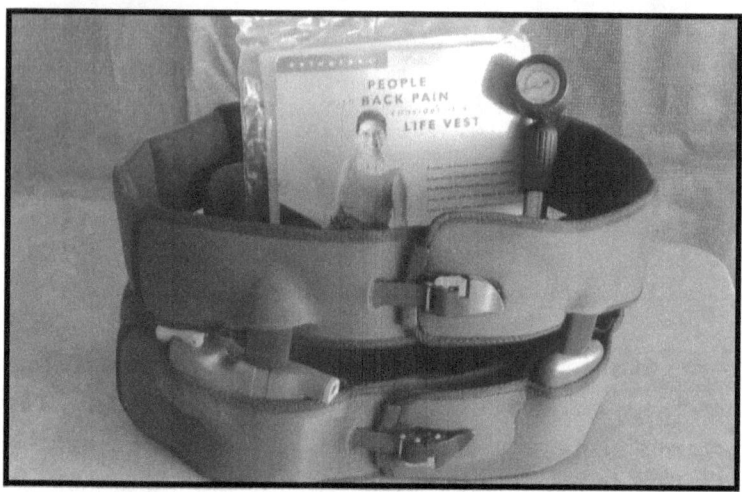

The new Orthotrac pneumatic vest effectively alleviates intervertebral compression and chronic pain. In fact associated leg pain is often relieved with minutes of application.

The Orthotrac is the only ambulatory treatment shown to decompress the spine using patented administered pneumatic lifting. The vest is designed to lift a weight of 50 to 30 percent of body weight from the lumbar spine onto the iliac crests.

TRUE DIRECTIONS
AN AFFILIATE OF TARCHER BOOKS

OUR MISSION

Tarcher's mission has always been to publish books
that contain great ideas. Why? Because:

GREAT LIVES BEGIN WITH GREAT IDEAS

At Tarcher, we recognize that many talented authors, speakers, educators,
and thought-leaders share this mission and deserve to be published
– many more than Tarcher can reasonably publish ourselves. True
Directions is ideal for authors and books that increase awareness, raise
consciousness, and inspire others to live their ideals and passions.

Like Tarcher, True Directions books are designed to do three things:
inspire, inform, and motivate.

Thus, True Directions is an ideal way for these important voices to
bring their messages of hope, healing, and help to the world.

Every book published by True Directions– whether it is non-fiction, memoir,
novel, poetry or children's book – continues Tarcher's mission to publish works
that bring positive change in the world. We invite you to join our mission.

For more information, see the True Directions website:
www.iUniverse.com/TrueDirections/SignUp

Be a part of Tarcher's community to bring positive change in this world!
See exclusive author videos, discover new and exciting books, learn about
upcoming events, connect with author blogs and websites, and more!
WWW.TARCHERBOOKS.COM

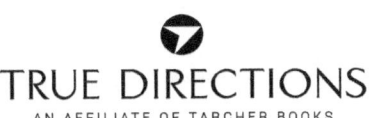

TRUE DIRECTIONS
AN AFFILIATE OF TARCHER BOOKS